© O Bruhn 2022

Table of Contents

S1. BACKGROUND..5
   1. Introduction..7
   2. Atavistic Regression & Stillness Meditation.....................11
   3. The Mind's Self Balancing Mechanism............................17

S2. MEARES' WORK ON CANCER..................................23
   4. Cancer Formation..25
   5. Stillness Meditation & Cancer.....................................29
   6. Individuals & Outcomes...39
   7. Onflow & Other Terms..45

S3. MEARES' MEDICAL PROTOCOL..............................49
   8. Becoming a Stillness Meditation Teacher 51
   9. Daily Preparation to Teach..55
   10. Initial Contact..57
   11. Greeting & Preliminary Meeting................................59
   12. Group Facilitation..63
   13. Bridging The Space Between....................................73
   14. Waking Up..79
   15. Separate From Stillness Meditation...........................81

S4. A MODERN NON-MEDICAL PROTOCOL..................85
   16. Same But Different..87
   17. Helping Clients Find You...89
   18. Greet, Meet & Facilitate...93
   19. Therapeutic Touch...99
   20. Venue Design & Selection......................................107
   21. A Digital Venue...113
   22. Interfacing With Other Methods..............................115

S5. PROVIDING A HEALTH SERVICE..........................119
   23. Meditation Teaching is a Health Service...................121
   24. Care & Feedback 125
   25. "Do Nots" & Reporting...131
   26. OHS, Insurance & Records.....................................137
   27. Fees & Sources of Advice......................................143

S6. AFTERWARDS..147
   28. Meares' Article Bibliography...................................149
   30. Ongoing Development Tips.....................................155

**Dr Ainslie Meares on Teaching Meditation.
Facilitating Stillness in others after you know Stillness well yourself.**

By Owen Bruhn. Author & Publisher.
ISBN 978-0-6481084-6-7
Cover and graphic design by Arlo Bruhn.

Dedication
To Dr Ainslie Meares who showed me Stillness and "wrote everything down". To all my teachers.

Acknowledgement
Thanks to those who disclosed recollections of Dr Meares, his classes or other classes.

Disclaimer
This book is intended for general information only. It must not be used as a substitute for learning in person from a qualified teacher trainer.

The author and the publisher cannot and do not accept any responsibility for any person attempting to apply information and methods presented herein. The reader takes on complete responsible for applying information and methods in this book. This reader responsibility includes, but is not limited to, all responsibility both for themselves, others they attempt to teach and for third parties not limited to family and carers.

This book does not outline all applicable standards and laws. Nor does it outline all measures needed to comply. The reader must seek legal advice and make regular checks with all applicable jurisdictional authorities.

Copyright
© Owen Bruhn 2022. Except as provided by the Copyright Act 1968, no part of this publication may be reproduced, communicated to the public without the prior written permission of the copyright owner.

Poems are reproduced from the following poetry books written by Ainslie Meares, MD: A Way of Doctoring; Cancer Another Way; Dialogue on Meditation; Let's Be At Ease; Prayer and Beyond.

© O Bruhn 2022

S1. Background

1. Introduction

You invite me
To go into meditation,
To a strange country
Where I have not been before.

Without a journey
Into something new
You stay where you are
Like so many others.[1]

In your search, to learn, experience and teach deeper meditation you have come to read this book. Few books discuss the teaching of meditation. So, reading this book is to your advantage. Yet, to get the most out of it, one must first learn Dr Ainslie Meares' Stillness Meditation – this is an unavoidable precondition for teaching it. Those learning it will get far more out of <u>Ainslie Meares on Meditation</u>. A great many people, from all over the world, wrote to Ainslie Meares, MD saying that they had great help learning Stillness Meditation after reading one of his best-selling books. That book forms part of <u>Ainslie Meares on Meditation</u>.

Some people call what they do "stillness meditation" yet it almost certainly differs from Dr Meares' method. Additions and unnecessary complexity prevent the Still mind state that is so important in both learning and teaching Dr Meares' method. A huge elephant in the room that remains invisible to many people.

Dr Meares trained in psychiatry and become an internationally recognised medical hypnotist. He transitioned to exclusively teaching Stillness Meditation as it was more effective than hypnotic techniques (including some he had invented). Meares' writings on teaching are scattered throughout his 36 books and many papers. The 2020-2023 pandemic stopped meditation teaching in Victoria. So, locked down with a PC and Meares' works, I wrote this book.

---

1 Meares A. Dialogue on Meditation. 1979. p7

An Overview Of This Book

S1. Background

First, there is background on hypnosis, atavistic regression and Ainslie Meares' Stillness Meditation. After that is discussion of Meares' ideas about the minds self balancing mechanism that allows Stillness and operates in all effective mental therapy. The evolutionary context of this self balancing mechanism is discussed.

S2. Cancer

Meares refined his ideas on atavistic regression during his last phase and these are explained from the perspective of the **non-medical** meditation teacher.

S3. Meares' Protocol

Section 3 contains Meares' medical meditation teaching protocol. Personal observations of mine and others are often but not always footnoted. Some seem less important or too obvious to bother footnoting. Footnoting, like citation, tends to reduce readability.

The term "meditation teacher" is so well-known it continues to be used here. Yet, it is more accurate to describe teaching Meares' Stillness Meditation as **facilitation**. Facilitation is unlike teaching science or maths in the classroom.

Just as Stillness Meditation is a unified experience so is facilitating it. Here, as Meares' explained it in his writings, the facilitation process is artificially broken down into pieces. Yet, it is an organic holistic process. A book about it can be read alongside a live course or as professional development. You can learn a lot from a book. Yet, reading can't replace the fluid organic experience.

Meares' **medical** meditation teaching protocol was based on a close doctor-**patient** relationship. The term **client** is used when discussing the non-medical equivalent.

S4. A Modern Non-Medical Protocol

I undertook systems analyses and design whilst working as an occupational health practitioner and trainer. S4 provides tips and insights from these methodologies.

An earlier draft of S3 had Meares' protocol mixed in with later material. To ensure transparency, the later material was excised and became S4.

The more I learn about Meares' protocol, the more I support the use of wanted appropriate soothing touch after informed consent. Sadly, in modern times, touch is fraught. The reader will need to carefully consider their own situation and weigh up the risks and benefits of the use of touch.

S5. Providing a Health Service

Dr Meares' taught within a doctor-**patient** framework. Modern meditation teachers provide a health service to **clients.** Attempting to incorporate this health service framework into an earlier draft of Meares' protocol only added complication. Instead, general principles of the health services framework are discussed in S5 based upon my experience working in the public and private sector. S5 was written in Victoria in 2022. Checks by the reader are needed as applicable laws and standards on meditation teaching vary by location, change over time, and professional bodies, insurers and regulators may each hold their own interpretation as to applicability and compliance. The best check is an informed legal opinion. If you operate outside of Australia always check with your local authorities.

S6. Afterwards

Footnoted references are used quite a lot in S2 (on Cancer) and S5 (on the health services framework). In other Sections, footnoted references were more restricted as they hindered communication. In S6, a complete bibliography of Meares' articles is shared (Ch. 28). Papers particularly relevant to teaching and cancer are flagged. A Key to the Books of Ainslie Meares provides a bibliography of Meares' books. The book concludes with some tips on ongoing development(Ch. 30).

The pandemic stopped meditation teaching in Victoria and so I distilled Ainslie Meares' ideas on teaching into this new book. I hope to substantially upgrade this work over time.

Owen Bruhn, 2023

2. Atavistic Regression & Stillness Meditation

Atavistic Regression

Meares became involved in hypnosis in 1947[2]. He published 16 papers between 1954-1956. 17 papers formed his Doctoral Dissertation. The last paper[3] in his dissertation concluded that hypnosis involved a simple mental state in which the mind atavistically regressed (ie. regressed to a state similar to that of a remote primitive ancestor). In that state, logical and critical faculties were absent, suggestion was pronounced with various overlay or phenomena present. Atavistic regression explained the many features of hypnosis which earlier theories had failed to explain.

In his 1956 Beattie-Smith Lecture[4], Meares outlined the history of hypnosis starting in the Paleolithic era. *"In primitive cultures, hypnosis is seen in the trance state of ritual and initiation" "mystery still surrounds the sacred sleep of the ancient Egyptian temples but it is believed that the priests [induced] hypnotic sleep....as a balm for... distress" "the practice of auto-hypnosis was organised into a philosophical system... "it found expression in Sanskrit in the Yoga Sutras of Patanjali... this system aims at spiritual liberation through sensory withdrawal and meditation. It has religious, philosophical and medical components..."*

Later in the same lecture, Meares notes: *" a doctor in India, Esdaile by name carried out a number of surgical operations under hypnosis without pain to the patient... There is no doubt as to authenticity.. "*

In the 1840s, a British Surgeon, James Esdaile[5] had carried out about 300 surgical operations under hypnosis without pain and these had been verified and were beyond doubt. Esdaille's work, as

---

2 Meares A (1967) Proc Medico-Legal Society Vict V11: 73-84.
3 Meares A (1957) AMA Archiv Neurol & Psychiatry, 77(5): 549-55. Published just after Meares' dissertation was submitted.
4 Meares A (1956) Med J Aust 1(1):1-5.
5 Esdaile J. Mesmerism in India, and its practical application in surgery and medicine. 1846. Reprinted in 1976 by Longman, London; Atkinson J & O'Shaughnessy (1847) Edinburgh Medical & Surgical J. 67(171): 581-588. *Report of Committee appointed by Bengal Government to examine Esdaile's work.*

Meares pointed out, had been overlooked due to the arrival of chemical anaesthesia in Europe.

The 1956 lecture and his Doctoral Dissertation make clear that Meares would travel to Asia to make further observations regarding atavistic regression and pain control. He did so, 4 years later in 1960[6]. In 1959, he forecast his trip the following year: *"there have always been those who... have sought to avoid pain by... evoking an inhibitory function of the mind... some have inhibited it in the trance state of Yoga... Hypnotherapists and Yogis use the trance state to inhibit pain. Why can't we develop this inhibitory power of the mind, and use it in our everyday life?"*

Naturally, Meares' was not the only one who sought to know the relationship between various hypnotic, meditative and related states – sometimes referred to by others as supra-conscious experiences. In 1966, Meares[7] responded to a letter published in the American Journal of Psychiatry: *"My interest.. led me to ...investigate the phenomenon in conditions uncontaminated by western sophistication."* By this Meares referred to his many field trips on the way to and from medical conferences to meet with experts (Yoga, Zen, Sufi, fire-walkers, Macumba etc[8]). Meares continues: *"The bridge between... mysticism and... psychiatry, is of course hypnosis. In both we have the same regression... I have led patients into deep hypnosis by completely passive and almost nonverbal techniques. [Patients speak] of the experience in terms... consistent with supra-conscious experiences... [They show]... marked relief of symptoms and a subtle change of personality toward better integration and greater understanding."*[9]

Atavistic regression as a common factor. Meares believed that atavistic regression was a common factor in meditative, hypnotic, mystic and other trance states[10]. That does **not** mean that these states are identical, even in hypnosis there are different sub-states. Nor does it mean that the processes involved in reaching them are identical. There are differences.

Major differences between "conventional" hypnosis and Stillness Meditation are outlined below. Meares' atavistic regression theory of

---

6 *This date is corroborated in several of his books and papers written around then.*
7 Meares A (1966) Am J Psychiatry 122(8): 953-954.
8 Meares A. Strange Places Simple Truths. 1969..
9 Meares A (1966) Am J Psychiatry 122(8): 953-954.
10 Meares A (1961) In Proc 3rd World Congress of Psychiatry. Pp 712-4; Meares A (1969). Existential Psychiatry pp119-121; Meares A (1975).in Unestahl LE (Ed). VIth Int Congress for Hypnosis. Pp159-160.

mental homeostasis and categorisation of meditative states are discussed later (Ch. 3 & 5).

Induction of hypnosis. Hypnosis may be induced by many means as discussed extensively by Dr Meares himself in his 500 page textbook, A Medical System of Hypnosis and his dissertation.

Authoritative induction relies on the power, prestige and status of the hypnotist. The hypnotist becomes large and powerful as the subject becomes tiny and insignificant and is pushed or pulled into hypnosis. The related confusion techniques bamboozles the subject which pushes them into hypnosis[11].

Passive induction was a more recent development. It is used less as it is more work for the hypnotist. The hypnotist guides and supports the patient to allow themselves to drift into hypnosis. Rapport between patient and hypnotist is essential. Passive induction is closely related to facilitation of Stillness Meditation.

Auto-hypnosis is taught by hypnotising the subject several times and giving them cues they use on themselves. Auto-hypnosis has an obvious relationship with meditation.

Depth of hypnosis. Earlier in his career, Meares had learnt how to hypnotise patients so deeply they ceased talking. They could hold a pen and so, he had them draw or paint. Due to the depth of hypnosis some experienced "catalepsy" (loss of voluntary motion) and couldn't hold the pen. So, Meares gave them clay, and they were able to model the thing in their minds that was distressing them. Meares' ability to achieve great depth of hypnosis is critical to understanding why his findings differed from those of some others. For example, some hypnotists state that only a proportion of subjects can be hypnotised. However, with rapport and the dynamic method (below). Meares found all subjects could undergo hypnosis.

The dynamic method. Many hypnotists used just one method of induction. They applied the same method rigidly to every patient. Meares' developed a flexible approach in which he used all the available methods and altered his approach "second by second" depending on the needs and response of the patient as the process unfolded. Hence, it was a dynamic method of hypnosis[12]. It was this flexible approach, together with depth, that enabled Meares to identify the best methods: *"Patients were making spectacular recoveries... Then an unexpected disillusionment came... the patients were getting well too quickly... By reducing my hypnotic procedures to greater and greater simplicity, I have been able to show that the effective mechanism... lies in the hypnosis itself, and*

---

[11] Meares A (1962) in Schneck JM (Ed) Hypnosis in Modern Medicine pp390–405.
[12] Meares A (1955) Med J Aust 1(18): 644-6.

not in the disclosure of the unconscious conflicts."[13] From then onwards, he showed patients how to let themselves pass into the Still mind state as he believed this was most effective.

Differences of Stillness Meditation from conventional hypnosis. In passive hypnosis, the hypnotist guides and supports, which is close to facilitation of Stillness Meditation although aspects of the induction may differ. Stillness Meditation is under the complete **voluntary** control of the client. The teacher's calm helps the client pass into the Still mind state. Both hypnosis and Stillness Meditation involve temporary atavistic regression. In Stillness Meditation, the regression continues to the still mind state. In other hypnotic and meditative states phenomena or mental activity (eg."thinking", sensory or emotional activity) continues (see Ch. 5)[14].

The Process of Stillness Meditation

Over time, Dr Meares simplified his explanation of Stillness Meditation as much as he could. Noting that the process of Stillness Meditation involves parts of the mind, where words do not live. Stillness Meditation is based on:

- Progressive relaxation
- Experiencing relaxation so it spreads throughout all of ourself, so our whole being is globally relaxed.
- Practised in slight discomfort.

In Stillness of the mind our brain is able to integrate the excessive input. Mental equilibrium is restored and anxiety is reduced. Perhaps, two more points might be made:

- Voluntary global relaxation leads to Stillness of mind.
- The teacher facilitates but, the client remains "in charge".

Physical relaxation. The first stage, complete physical relaxation of the body, is an all embracing experience. Some people may think to use progressive muscular relaxation to learn the feeling of relaxing muscles. However, in progressive relaxation the mind is alert and this prevents Stillness. A mind that is alert is not relaxed. Progressive relaxation must shift into global relaxation.

Experience the relaxation. The second step is to learn to experience the relaxation so it spreads throughout our whole self. The body is relaxed and this expands into the mind. Our mind experiences the mental equivalent of bodily relaxation. The mind slows. Not all at once. It slows and stills momentarily. Then this

---

13 Meares A (1971) Aust J Forensic Sci 3(4): 157-161.
14 Meares A (1968). Int J Clin Exp Hyp. 16(4):211-4; Meares A (1978). J Am Soc Psych Dent Med 25(4):129-32.

happens for longer periods. We know of the Stillness afterwards.

Slight discomfort. The third step is to meditate in slight discomfort. As we have discussed, relaxation can come from the body and the mind. Relaxation of just the body does not help the mind. Laying on a bed, or slumped comfortably on a padded sofa, one feels bodily relaxed from nerve impulses from limb and trunk that report their physical relaxed state. There is no mentally therapeutic effect from meditating in comfort. This can only occur in relaxation that comes from our mind. In a slightly uncomfortable position our mind transcends the discomfort, and we are no longer aware of it. Not too much discomfort though, to avoid tensing up.

Calm And Ease In Daily Life

After the finish, there is a deep calm. This persists for periods of varying lengths. With practice this after-meditation calm becomes longer until, eventually, it becomes a part of every day life - living a calm and active life.

Meares' method is more than meditation! More than learning to meditate. Calm and ease in daily living is the sine qua non (ie. "that without which it is not"). Learning to let the after-meditation calm carry over into the rest of the day is the main part of the equation.

Practising Stillness Meditation without letting the effects of it carry over into daily life is far less effective. We do not live to meditate. We meditate to live a better life. An active life with a calm mind and body. Together with ease in action and response.

Calm. Confidence. Courage. Contentment. If we are tense, behaviours that reduce short term stress also tend to increase longer term stress (and or depression etc). For example, avoiding a situation that might stress also results in the reward staying out of reach. Reducing stress helps us to cope better with such situations. It enables us to take (sensible) actions rather than avoiding as we may have done in the past.

"Calmness leads to confidence. Confidence leads to courage. Courage means facing life challenges, meeting those challenges and being rewarded with success - and then achievement ... and adventure ... and little by little... that leads to Contentment. And so life gets better, and better."[15]

Over the page, one of Meares' poems concludes this Chapter.

---

15 McKinnon P (2018) A calm mind and a beautiful life! Stillness Meditation Therapy Centre Blog July 2018.

The meditation
Of a way of doctoring
Is very simple,
Very simple indeed;
Like the thoughts and feelings of a child,
So simple,
So difficult
For adults to comprehend.

No forcing ourself
No striving to do it
No contemplation of any image
No awareness of our breathing
No repetition of a mantra
No forcing ourself to maintain a posture.

Just slightly uncomfortable
Just slightly so
We let go
And we are no longer aware
Of the slight discomfort.

Not asleep
Not fully consciousness
Mind is clear
We experience a profound state
Of heavenly naturalness,
Just the act of being.[16]

---

16 Meares A. A Way of Doctoring. 1984. No 38 , pg18

© O Bruhn 2022

3. The Mind's Self Balancing Mechanism

"The most important thing we can do in helping our brain integrate the excess of impulses which it is receiving is to let our mind run quietly for a while. This not only temporarily reduces the overload on our brain, but actually helps our brain to work more effectively."[17]

Why People Get Better

Why do people with nervous illness get better? A fundamental question. It was one that Dr Ainslie Meares[18] pondered for years.

A few people recover spontaneously from nervous illness. Their environment remains unchanged. So, this must be a result of some internal readjustment.

Others improve as a result of a lessening of external stress (ie. their environment has changed). Or, some therapeutic experience in their life situation has occurred.

Some lose their symptoms in circumstances without a therapist-patient relationship. Examples of this can include medication, rest and prayer. Even the rest from a holiday sometimes results in a loss of nervous symptoms.

Those with a therapist-patient relationship may lose their symptoms after many types of treatment. These include a quiet talk with the family doctor, tranquillisers, simple psychotherapy, abreaction, conditioning, waking suggestion, hypnotic treatment etc.

Dr Meares concluded that there must be **a common factor** involved in all these situations. Nervous illness involves an upset. So, a self adjusting mechanism of the mind is able to restore balance if the correct circumstances are provided. This self balancing mechanism is involved in all successful treatments. It was Meares' "*Atavistic Regression Theory of Mental Homeostasis*".

A plain language description of Meares theory is provided below. This plain version simplifies it a bit, after that is a detailed description from one of Meares' medical text books.

The Mind's Self Balancing System

Stress can arise from the mind, body or external environment.

---
17 Meares A. Life Without Stress. 1987.
18 *Meares' thoughts summarised from 1961-1962 Lancet articles in Ch 28.*

One or more such stresses may flood the mind's integrating mechanism. This is felt as anxiety. A warning signal.

Normally, **the self balancing mechanism** restores balance. This is more difficult if:
- The re-balancing pattern wasn't learned properly as a child.
- Internal conflicts related to the stressful situation add extra stress. The patient is unaware of these unconscious internal conflicts. They feel stress which may seem out of proportion to the situation.

If stress is severe, and or prolonged, then it results in ongoing anxiety as the self balancing mechanism is unable to restore balance.

Anxiety is a warning signal. It produces an alerting response. This includes the sympathetic nervous system gearing up for danger. Preparation for physical "**fight or flight**" is inappropriate for an internal threat as motion is not required. Hence, sympathetic nervous system overactivity can't be dissipated. The nervous system compensates but stays out of balance. This is why bodily symptoms may result from either sympathetic or parasympathetic overactivity. For example, gut symptoms can be a response to stress. If stress related gut symptoms occur, diarrhoea is often related to acute stress and a parasympathetic "overshoot" into constipation may occur later.

In other cases, psychological "conversion" may relieve anxiety by producing bodily symptoms. This conversion to bodily symptoms provides a symbolic solution that reduces anxiety.

Anxiety is relieved by any procedure that aids the self balancing mechanism. This element is present in all medical and non-medical procedures that reduce anxiety. Such treatments are only effective when accompanied by operation of this self balancing mechanism.

Normally, the level of mental function fluctuates. Sometimes, an individual is alert, logical and critical. At other times, they are relaxed and uncritical. They may drift into restful reverie. Like sleep, these moments of spontaneous slowing (and sometimes stilling) of the mind allow the self balancing mechanism to restore and maintain mental balance. Such moments might be thought of as brief spontaneous Stillness Meditation sessions. Meares' approach was to ensure that adequate time is spent in mental Stillness by formal practice sessions 10-15 minutes twice daily.

The patient with chronic anxiety keeps their guard up. They can no longer let it down and don't show a normal fluctuation in the level of mental function. The management of the anxious patient facilitates periods of slowing and stilling of the mind. All treatments for anxiety must always allow for this concurrent experience.

Meares' Describes His Theory

Meares published several descriptions of his atavistic regression theory of mental homeostasis. The one below, from Meares' textbook, *Management Of The Anxious Patient*[19], provides an excellent overview.

"*Stress from intrapsychic, bodily or environmental influences may result in sensory input which floods the integrating mechanism of the mind. The subject then becomes aware of this disordered function as the experience of anxiety, which thus works as a warning signal that all is not well.*

In ordinary circumstances the homeostatic mechanism comes into play and restores psychic equilibrium. If a pattern for the easy re-establishment of equilibrium has not been learned in infancy and childhood, or if unconscious conflicts in the same area add to the present stress, homeostasis becomes more difficult. If stress is of sufficient severity, and if it is sufficiently prolonged, the homeostatic mechanism may be unable to restore equilibrium, and the subject suffers from an anxiety state.

Because anxiety acts as a warning that all is not well, it produces an alerting response in which the sympathetic-adrenal system is activated in preparation to meet the threatened emergency. This preparation, for motor activity is an inappropriate response for the stress situation, which is an internal rather than an external threat. The sympathetic overactivity cannot be dissipated in effective action. In order to restore equilibrium in the autonomic system, compensatory parasympathetic activity is evoked. In this way psychosomatic symptoms may result from either sympathetic or parasympathetic overactivity.

On the other hand psychological mechanisms may come into play to relieve the anxiety by producing hysterical bodily symptoms (ie a conversion disorder), which provides a symbolic solution for the patient's conflict. With the stress situation resolved in this symbolic way, the patient is relatively free from anxiety.

The anxiety state may be relieved by any procedure that is effective in aiding the function of the homeostatic mechanism, and is a constant factor in all medical and non-medical procedures effective in allaying anxiety.

Therapeutic mechanisms such as conditioning, suggestion, insight, and rapport are effective when they operate on a basis of

---

19 Meares A. Management Of The Anxious Patient.1963. P42-43 which form Ch. 6. and titled "Statement of the atavistic theory". *Reading makes clear that Ch. 6 in that 493 page book is a summary of Ch.5 pp29-41.* .

atavistic regression. But unless they are accompanied by atavistic regression these potentially therapeutic mechanisms are ineffective.

The individual in normal health is subject to constant fluctuations in the level of his mental functioning. Sometimes he is alert, logical and critical. At other times he is relaxed and uncritical, and occasionally he drifts into reverie. Like sleep, these moments of spontaneous atavistic regression are necessary if the homeostatic mechanism is to maintain psychic equilibrium. The patient with chronic anxiety state remains constantly on guard and no longer shows normal fluctuations in his level of mental functioning.

Our management of the anxious patient must be so ordered as to facilitate periods of atavistic regression, and our technique of using conditioning, suggestion, insight and rapport must always allow for concurrent atavistic regression".

In Meares' Stillness Meditation the body and mind relax. The mind slows down and becomes still. Tension and anxiety cannot exist when the mind is still. There is an absence of disturbance and profound mind-body rest. Afterwards, the mind feels calm. Sometimes, the calm is profound. Even tranquil or serene. Some might call it equanimity. However, equanimity can have an incorrect connotation of blunting or lacking emotional sensitivity, which is harmful. It is not that. Rather, an absence of disturbance, natural mental rest, integration, and the restoration of balance.

How Homeostasis by Regression Evolved[20]

Some assume that meditation involves a higher, superior mental state. Like the step from animal to human mind they see it as a next step that takes the adherent to something beyond human. However, evolution can work in other ways. It always proceeds from stable to newer function. Stability can enable a new function or state to work better. Sometimes, stability involves a step back to regain balance in order to step forwards and upwards.

In the evolution of animals, there was a time before consciousness. A long, long time ago, a distant ancestor advanced and consciousness evolved. However, these conscious animals periodically returned to unconsciousness. There were cycles of unconsciousness (sleep) and waking. Various emotions subsequently emerged, early ones included the fight-flight response and also feeding and resting.

A million years before humans existed, primitives no longer ape,

---

20 Refer Appendix 1, Still Mind Sound Body

but not much more than that, had minds that were "empty" as they could not think. Much later, our early Homo Sapiens ancestors began to think. Thinking was new. Initially, there were problems "jumping up" into the new thinking state. A less obvious problem was that thinking allowed high levels of anxiety to build up. Some early ones jumped and got stuck thinking, became highly anxious or even went mad. Eventually, some began to experience fluctuation in their waking state. There were times when their minds went off guard, and they lapsed into a sort of reverie. A day-dream without the dream, as such. A temporary return to the waking state of ancestors unable to think. A state that provided natural mental rest and relieved anxiety. Periods of thinking interspersed with mental rest. This seems similar to evolution's earlier solution of waking and sleep. The recipe of adequate sleep and natural mental rest from Stillness Meditation being necessary for further evolution of the human mind.

Evolution & Teaching Meares' Meditation

Meditation involves communication between the teacher and client. Again, evolution is relevant although we need to go back only so far as our primitive ancestors or mammals.

Groups of mammals, whether predator or prey, depend upon others in the group. If all is quiet without danger, then the group tends to settle into grazing, resting or similar behaviours etc. However, if one in the group notices some potential danger (predator, enemy etc) then the group becomes alert. There is a survival advantage as the alerting response enables the group to react more quickly. However, the hyperdrive of the fight-flight response places short term survival ahead of medium-long term health. So, when threats are absent the group, under ordinary circumstances, relaxes into a "rest and digest" response. Under normal circumstances, the resting response prevailed much of the time. Until, a new threat alerted the more sensitive individuals, who alerted the group, so they were ready to fight or flee. After the threat was abolished the group returned to the resting state.

We have within us the ability to take on the mood of others. Many people are familiar with the ability of certain politicians and fanatics to whip a crowd into a violent frenzy ("herd poison" is an abusive degrading use of the crowd). However, less obvious, but far more important, is that people can communicate a state of passive calm to one another. There are some people who have an air of calm about them. Those who know them experience calm when in the company of that person.

The communication of calm from one to another is the basis of the teaching of Meares Stillness Meditation. It emphasise the importance of having learnt Meares' Stillness Meditation and being calm and at ease (outside of meditation) before starting to teach. It can be seen why facilitating is a better description than teaching.

If you want to go straight to Meares' protocol you can skip to Section 3 (Ch. 8) and return to the next Section (Section 2 on cancer) later on.

S2. Meares' Work On Cancer

4. Cancer Formation

Introduction

Some clients decide to take up Stillness Meditation as they are ill with a chronic disease such as cancer. A Stillness Meditation teacher is not a cancer doctor and can't provide medical advice. Yet, sick clients ask questions and need accurate information.

This section (S2) discusses:
- basic aspects of the process of cancer formation.
- how Stillness Meditation influences cancer (Ch. 5).
- individual and group outcomes. (Ch. 6).
- disentangling Meares' Onflow from terms used by some other people to help avoid confusion (Ch. 7).

Ainslie Meares' work on cancer also led him to fine-tuning his explanations of his method. Do read this section at some point as it will deepen your understanding of Meares' ideas. If you want to go straight to Meares' protocol you can skip to Section 3 (Ch. 8) and return to this Section later.

Willis' Definition

There are many definitions of cancer, however, one is needed that conveys the general idea rather than overwhelming technical detail. So, we turn to a long-standing definition provided by a pathologist named Willis[21] in 1960: "*an abnormal mass of tissue, the growth of which exceeds and is uncoordinated with that of the normal tissues, and persists in the same excessive manner after cessation of the stimuli which evoked the change.*"

Basic Factors in Cancer Formation

Growth. Cell division and growth are normal. Cells normally grow and divide. This occurs in the embryo, during childhood and on into maturity. If cell division and growth go wrong then that can cause a rogue cell that divides more than it should. The rogue cells offspring (rogue cell line) have genetic changes (damage) that allows or even encourages poorly controlled cell division. The rogues cell and its offspring might be thought of as pre-cancerous or on the way

---

21 Willis RA. Pathology of Tumours. 3rd ed. Butterworth. 1960. pg1002. *Willis's cancer definition included both benign & malignant tumours.*

to becoming a cancer.

Injury. Injury (chemical, physical, microbial etc) and inflammatory response can result in genetic changes and an environment that allow cells to go rogue.

Self correction. On the other hand, the body normally endeavours to self correct when things go wrong. Components of inflammation and healing are part of such systems. Unsurprisingly, it is normal for systems in the body to detect and kill rogue cells.

Balance. The balance between:
- rogue cell formation and proliferation, and
- detection and removal of rogue cells,

determine if some rogue cells evade detection and grow into a lump.

Changed balance. The risk of a cancerous lump occurring can be increased or reduced by a change in the balance.

One change in the balance, increasing risk, would be something that creates and increases the number of rogue cells. This includes substantial exposure to things such as asbestos, tobacco smoking, radiation and so on.

Another change in the balance would be something that reduces surveillance and killing of rogue cells. This includes a damaged or defective immune system. Sometimes called immunosuppression.

Stress, Cortisol, Immunity & Cancer

Next is a tour through some history of science to put Meares' work in context. If you don't want to go on this tour, then go to the conclusion at the end of this chapter.

Stress. In 1936, Selye[22] reported that lab rats damaged by agents such as exposure to cold, surgical injury, excessive muscular exercise, or substances suffered a typical syndrome. He named it general adaptation syndrome or GAS. GAS consisted of enlarged adrenal glands, atrophy of the thymus and lymphatic tissue, and ulcerations of stomach and duodenum. Selye said GAS was stress.

Engineers would say that the GAS lab rats were strained. The dose (or stress) makes the response (or strain). Despite this usage, Selye named it "stress". It is far too late to change it to "strain" or "strain response" now. We are stuck with Selyes' confusing term.

Cortisol. Selye's work focused interest on various hormone secreting organs like the adrenal glands. By 1950, Hench, Kendall & Reichstein extracted cortisol from the adrenal cortex and used it in the laboratory and clinic. Cortisol like drugs include cortisone,

---

22 Selye H (1936). A syndrome produced by diverse nocuous agents. Nature 138: (3479,Jul 4):32. Selye H (1950). Stress and the general adaptation syndrome. 4667:1384-92;

prednisolone and so on[23].

Cushing's Syndrome[24] was first described in 1912. Biopsy of the adrenal cortex (ie. where cortisol is made) from Cushing's patients shows increased microscopic activity[25]. Cortisol levels in serum, saliva, and urine are raised in Cushing's syndrome[26]. Patients with Cushing's Syndrome are at risk of severe infections and sepsis. This was well-known back then.

Invaders & Immunity. Imhotep (2600 BC)[27], an Egyptian Pharaoh, used a special poultice and cut into the cancer in an attempt to treat it. If the infection didn't kill the patient then sometimes the cancer shrunk. In 1893[28], Coley saw a patient who unexpectedly recovered from cancer after surviving a serious infection. He identified 38 reports written by other doctors who had previously observed this phenomenon. Later, Coley treated patients with a sterile microbial extract (ie. with killed bacteria in it) that he hoped would do the same thing. He observed that quite a few of those he treated lived much longer than expected. Some had much less help and some died. Coley's extract whilst crude was safer than the Egyptian technique. It seemed more effective than other treatments available then. Even so, Coley "fell out of favour" until long after his death in the mid 1930s.

Reviews published from 1946-1953, indicated that about half of Coley's cancer patients lived on more than 5 years after treatment with his extract[29]. A 50% cure rate was impressive.

---

23 Cortisone is a naturally-occurring corticosteroid (metabolite) also used as a pharmaceutical prodrug. Prednisolone is a human-made form of cortisol.
24 Bauer J (1950). The so-called Cushing's Syndrome, its History, Terminology and Differential Diagnosis. Acta Med Scand 137: 411-416.; Cushing H (1912). The Pituitary Body and Its Disorders. J.B. Lippincott
25 *Increased basophilia of cortical cells on H&E stained histological sections.*
26 *There is a large literature from the 1940s-1970 with much work since then.*
27 Hopton Cann SA, van Netten JP, van Netten C, Glover DW (2002). Spontaneous regression: a hidden treasure buried in time. Med Hypotheses. 58(2):115-9
28 Coley WB (1893). The treatment of malignant tumors by repeated inoculations of erysipelas. Amer J Med Sci. 105(5):487–510; McCarthy EF (2006). The toxins of William B. Coley and the treatment of bone and soft-tissue sarcomas. Iowa Orthop J 26: 154–158.
29 Nauts HD, Swift WE & Colery BL (1946). The treatment of malignant tumors by bacterial toxins as developed by the late William B. Coley. Cancer Res 6:205–6. Nauts HC, Fowler GA & Bogatko GH (1953). A review of the influence of bacterial infection and of bacterial products (Coley's toxins) on malignant tumors in man. Acta Medica Scand 145: Supplement 276; Nauts HC, McLaren JR (1990) Coley Toxins - The First Century. In Bicher HI, McLaren JR, Pigliucci GM (eds) Consensus on Hyperthermia for the 1990s. Advances Exp Med and Biol V267;

Jumping around a bit, back to 1909, Ehrlich[30] had proposed that rogue cells are common but, are killed by the immune system nearly all the time. There was a long delay of 48 years, until Sir MacFarlane Burnett[31] put forward a modified version of Ehrlich's idea. That is, that single cancer cells grew into tiny clumps that provoked an immune response that killed them leaving no traces. In 1959, Old and others[32] found that BCG vaccine (a microbial extract!) inhibited cancer growth in the lab. Strangely, there was no mention of Coley's work in Old's paper or the many similar studies. Stimulation of the immune system by "vaccination" to fight cancer continued to be researched and was widely known by 1970[33].

Conclusion

Now the historical tour is ended, and we get to the point. By the time Meares' began his work on cancer it was known that:
- Normally, the immune tissues detect and kill rogue cells before any hint of a visible lump.
- Severe, prolonged stress weakens the immune system so it is much less able to kill microbes or rogue cells.
- Stimulating the immune system can enhance rogue cell detection and killing.
- Stress raises cortisol and this weakens detection and killing of microbes and rogue cells.
- Reducing stress has the opposite effect.

It was all documented in medical textbooks years before Meares began his work on cancer. Meares' approach was also facilitated by his keen insight and decades of experience using Stillness Meditation to help patients. Quite simply, his approach was consistent with conventional medical thinking. Yet, some medical practitioners and oncologists opposed Meares' work. That has changed over time. Yet, even in 2022, there remain some who deny any role of psychological factors in cancer formation and treatment.

---

30 Ehrlich P. Über den jetzigen stand der karzinomforschung. Ned Tijdschr Geneeskd 1909; 5: 273-290.
31 Burnett FM, Cancer A biological approach. Br Med J.1957;1:779–782.
32 Old LJ, Clarke DA & Benacerraf B (1959). Effect of Bacillus Calmette Guerin infection on transplanted tumors in the mouse. Nature 1959 Jul 25; 184: 291-292.
33 Morton DL, Eilber FR, Joseph WL, et al (1970). Immunological factors in human sarcomas and melanomas. Ann Surg Oct; 172: 740-49 ; Morales A, Eidinger D & Bruce AW (1976). Intracavitary Bacillus Calmette-Guerin in the treatment of superficial bladder tumors. J Urol. 116(2):180-3.

5. Stillness Meditation & Cancer

Introduction

It first occurred to Dr Ainslie Meares that Stillness Meditation might influence cancer just after World War II (ie. after 1945)[34].

In the 1950s[35] & '60s, he taught patients Stillness Meditation to reduce the hurt from pain due to cancer. They learnt to manage pain and some had an unexpected side effect. The growth of the cancer slowed. Much later, looking back over his life's work Meares[36] wrote:

> This was my dream.
> Like so many dreams
> Day followed day,
> And year followed year
> Before I could muster the courage
> To test it
> In the cold light of reality.

In the mid 1970s, Meares saw a few cancer patients near death and for whom there was no other treatment. They benefited enough that he continued his work and wrote many papers on the effect of Stillness Meditation on cancer (Ch. 28 lists them). **Four factors** were important:
1. A profound and prolonged reduction in the level of anxiety.
2. A physiological regression to the state that prevailed before the cancer.
3. Healing, which is a primitive function involving regression.
4. A type of meditation involving Stillness of the mind.

Only, Stillness Meditation met all these requirements.

Later, each of the 4 factors are discussed in turn. But, first a quote from an article Meares wrote in the Lancet[37] several years after he had begun his work on cancer: "... *the time has come for doctors to seriously to investigate the psychological approach to*

---
34 Meares A. A Way of Doctoring. 1984. pp112-113.
35 Meares A. A Better Life. 1989. p113.
36 Meares A. A Way of Doctoring. 1984. pg113.
37 Meares A (1981) Lancet 2(8254):1037-1038.

cancer...We should be prepared to face inevitable criticism... We must be prepared for some kind of reaction on the part of the profession similar to that experienced by those who first attempted to relieve organic symptoms of gross hysteria by psychological means."

Some 25 years earlier, Meares had lectured on the history of hypnosis from Stone Age times right up until 1956[38]. In this lecture he described how prominent hypnotists of the 1800s like Mesmer, Esdaille, Braid, Elliotson etc. *"attempted to relieve organic symptoms of gross hysteria".* They all became outcasts whose contributions were not fully recognised during their lifetimes. In modern times, it is popular to question the meaning of words like hysteria. Some people misunderstand "hysteria". Hysteria, in the sense Meares' used it, meant bodily symptoms arising from "anxiety conversion" reactions (see later) in humans of both sexes[39]. Anxiety conversion reactions have nothing to do with wandering wombs as such[40]. Irony is heaped upon irony as these conversion reactions are involved in some (but not all!) cancers. More on that later.

A profound and prolonged reduction in anxiety is the first of the 4 factors.

Anxiety & Cancer

Emotion & Cancer

Inducing cancer in the laboratory involves a convenient external agent (like a chemical or physical agent). This approach can tend to overlook the role of emotional factors. Yet, Selye's work (Ch. 4) made it clear that stress must be involved in cancer formation. Meares noted that medical writers from 1700- 1800s, reported negative emotional states were often associated with cancer. He referred to Le Shan[41] whose review of negative emotional states and cancer commenced with the Roman physician, Galen. There is not the space to discuss it all here, but there was a lot of it.

Marked stress 6-24 months before diagnosis. Over time Meares saw many cancer patients. He observed that all of them had experienced a prolonged and difficult source of stress. This related to an unsolvable problem in the period, 6 months to 2 years, leading

---

38 *See, for example:* Meares A. (1956) Med J Aust 1(1):1-5 & 1(2):37–40.
39 *Refer* Management of the Anxious Patient *for full details.*
40 *The Egyptians thought that the womb might be shifted by disease or back to its correct position by treatment. The term "hysteria" comes from an Ancient Greek word for womb. Its technical meaning changed over time.*
41 Le Shan L (1959). Psychological Factors in the development of malignant disease. J Nat Cancer Inst 22:1-18

up to their diagnosis. Again, this confirmed the earlier findings of Le Shan[42]. The difficult problem may not have been obvious to the patient but, it was always present.

High anxiety suppressed the immune system. Meares believed that anxiety about the unsolvable problem raised cortisol (and other changes) that suppressed the immune system. This reduced its ability to kill cancer cells.

Conversion Reactions

Anxiety "conversion". Over decades, Meares had seen that many conditions resulting from anxiety were helped by learning Stillness Meditation. Some of them were completely eliminated.

In his work, after World War 2, he saw the full range of severe anxiety reactions amongst traumatised military personnel. In some cases, the anxiety was severe enough that the mind controlled the body. For example, sometimes a soldier stumbled and tripped or fell. They found they could not get up as a leg.was paralysed. They could not walk, and so could not go towards the battle! Of course, not all cases of limb paralysis are due to anxiety about death. Damage to nerves and or joints etc. can result in irreversible paralysis of a limb.

Yet, sometimes a mind filled with horrendous anxiety found a way out by paralysing the limb. Of course, the mind also protected the soldier by pushing its "solution" down into the murky depths. Walling it off, so that there was no conscious awareness of it. All the soldier knew was that their leg.would not work as they couldn't make it move. The war had ceased but, paralysis was an ongoing problem for the soldier. Unless treated it was permanent even though there were no more battles. Early in his career, Meares had used deep hypnosis to remove limb paralysis caused by anxiety about death. This undoubtedly left a deep impression on both patient and practitioner.

Limb paralysis is one example of a "conversion" reaction. Another is the soldier who sees their mate(s) consumed by fire. Although further away, the soldier sees a flash and then nothing. Blinded, they can see no more horrible sights.

Conversion reactions, like limb paralysis and blinding, solve the short term problem. One soldier can't walk to the battle. Another can't see the aftermath. These symbolic solutions result in a substantial reduction in anxiety. Of course, the "side effects", paralysis or blindness, creates many ongoing problems in the activities of living.

Some cancer patients had a conversion reaction. Meares saw that, sometimes, cancer might involve a conversion reaction.

---

42 Le Shan L (1959). *as per just mentioned footnote.*

Some patients sought to escape from a horrible unsolvable problem through death. When stuck in a double bind, parts of the mind these patients had no conscious awareness of sought death as an escape. After the conversion of anxiety into symbolic solution, such patients would be expected to have a low level of anxiety. Meares observed that some of his cancer patients were like that. When they came to see him, they were dying yet, had an air of indifference about them (eg. it didn't matter as it would soon come to an end).

Dangers of discussion. The symbolic "escape by death" is pushed deep into the unconscious and walled off to protect the person from an acute breakdown. Any leakage through to consciousness may precipitate hostility even violent abreaction[43]. It is safer to provide a very general explanation that anxiety can contribute to cancer.

Psychosomatic Reactions

Meares observed that many cancer patients had high levels of anxiety. This was inconsistent with a conversion reaction. It was consistent with severe prolonged stress due to an unsolvable problem. In these patients, cancer was a psychosomatic illness. In other words, the immune suppression from high anxiety had allowed the cancer to develop. In other cases some external factor (eg. asbestos etc) increased damage that had increased rogue cell formation with reduced immune suppression due high anxiety.

Meares wrote: *We no longer expect to find a single cause for a disease; rather we expect to find a multiplicity of factors...it seems that reactions resembling those of psychosomatic illness and conversion* (reactions)*... operate as causes of cancer, more so in some cases than others, and that they operate in conjunction with the known chemical, viral and radiation causes of the disease.*[44]

Reducing Anxiety Always Helps

If the cause of severe prolonged stress is reduced, then the immune suppression is reduced or removed. This occurs regardless of the cause.

Stillness Meditation reduces anxiety. This helps the patient's immune system detect and kill the cancer cells. If there is a profound and prolonged reduction in the level of anxiety (see later) then the improvement becomes substantial over the fullness of time. This completes our discussion of the first element on Meares' list.

---

43 *see "Abreaction" in* Meares A (1963) Management of the Anxious Patient.
44 Meares A. (1981) The Lancet. Nov 7, 2(8254).1037-1038.

Regression & Healing

Relevant aspects of the atavistic regression hypothesis of mental homeostasis are further discussed below.

Physiological Regression

If an aspect of the body is working incorrectly then there must be a return to normality for it to work correctly. What has gone wrong must be "erased". There must be a physiological regression. A going backwards to the state before development of the maladaptive reaction. This regression lets the body's self-regulating mechanisms re-establish an appropriate pattern. The slate must be wiped clean before a better adaptive reaction can be put into place.

Atavistic regression facilitates both:
- removal of the maladaptive reaction, and
- the re-establishment of an appropriate pattern.

Long duration Stillness Meditation is needed to facilitate a physiological regression that wipes the slate clean and puts a better pattern into place. Physiological regression is particularly important for conversion reactions. It is also important for certain non-cancerous chronic conditions.

Healing

Sleep involves a loss of consciousness and represents a return towards the simpler state of mind that applied to distant ancestors before they had developed consciousness. The need for adequate sleep is well known. Those who are chronically sleep deprived may be unaware of their second class living until they get sufficient sleep.

Healing is also a primitive function of animals. The temporary "going backwards" to a simpler ancestral state (atavistic regression) meets this consideration.

Stillness & Other Types of Meditation

"Non-Still" States And Cancer Growth

Meares had taught a patient Stillness Meditation[45]. They had substantially improved ie. there was a marked shrinkage of the lump. Then, Meares went on annual leave. With Meares' absent, the patient decided that they could make Stillness Meditation more effective! They thought to visualise immune cells attacking the rogue cells in their mind's eye. The patient's condition rapidly deteriorated. On his return, Meares' re-established the patient's experience of Stillness and the cancer shrunk again. Clearly, the type of meditation is an important factor in the healing of cancer.

---

45 Meares A (1977). Med J Aust 2(4):132-133

Four Types Of Meditation

Decades earlier, Meares had described the various states of hypnosis[46]. Whilst the layperson thinks of hypnosis as a single state, there are several hypnotic states, for example, sleeping, abreaction and waking hypnosis. Now, Meares' work on cancer led him to categorise the types of meditation as follows:[47]

1. "Thought" based (eg. contemplating, examining, wandering).
2. Sensory based (eg. visualisation).
3. Emotion based (eg. compassion).
4. Meares' Stillness Meditation (aka mental ataraxis, see later).

In types 1-3, various combinations of the senses, emotions, intellect and will ("thought") are active. The persistence of phenomena (ie sensing, emotion etc) inhibit Stillness. For example, a visualising mind can't be still due to activity of the mind's eye. Similarly for both meditation-hypnotic induction using candle, bright light gazing or the fixed stare. The absence of visual sensation, indeed of sensation, emotion and "thought" is needed for Stillness to occur.

Meares' theory states that in types 1-3 meditation atavistic regression occurs with **phenomena present** (also the feelings associated with regression). Stillness cannot exist unless phenomena are absent.

The Fourth Type: Meares' Stillness Meditation

In the fourth type, Stillness Meditation, there is little or no mental activity as the mind is still (ie. neither "thought", sensation nor emotion). In other words, atavistic regression with a lack of mental activity results in mental ataraxis. **Ataraxis,** from the Greek, referring to a state with an absence of disturbance or equanimity.

If the effortless lessening of mental activity after atavistic regression continues then the person who remains awake, not asleep nor unconscious will experience mental ataraxis. By necessity, it is literally only lessening, leading to an absence of mental activity, that results in the Stillness aka mental ataraxis. Ataraxis cannot occur unless there is effortlessness that allows transcendence of slight discomfort. Slight discomfort is necessary to stay awake and so the mind participates in the relaxation. The mental lessening of effortless relaxation allows slowing that terminates in stillness. Both effortlessness and transcended slight discomfort must be present otherwise ataraxis can't occur.

---

46 Meares A. A System of Medical Hypnosis. 1960.
47 Meares A (1978) J Am Soc Psych Dent Med 25(4):129-32. *Meares categorised methods of meditation popular at the time. His skeletal framework is outlined here.*

© O Bruhn 2022

Relationship Between Regression & Ataraxis

Meares writes that only mental ataraxis was able to provide the conditions needed to help heal cancer. Throughout his writings, Hypnotic, meditative and other trance states involve an atavistic regression with phenomena or overlay present.[48] Mental ataraxis only occurs when phenomena are absent.

A meditator (type 1-3) who has atavistically regressed and effortlessly lessens mental activity might then pass into mental ataraxis\Stillness. Given that clinging to phenomena inhibits ataraxis it would be luck rather than method design per se. Lucky slips may occur if practice occurs over a very long timeframe ie. years or longer. On the other hand, Meares' simple, direct and efficient approach is to relax, allow the mind to slow down and become still. This needs practice sessions of relatively short duration over a relatively short learning period (ie for learning vs. healing cancer). It is outside the experience of other methods.

Meares wrote that some people who practised other types of meditation come to see him for help. They were examples[49] of where things had gone wrong. Meares' helped them to put things right. For example, some who had practised breath counting couldn't stop the inner counter in their mind's ear. They had to unlearn inner counting in learning to let the mind still. Similarly, others were distressed when they found their mind persistently uttered a mantra and would not stop. In another example, some "focusing" on the present moment found obsessive mental checking became distressing. Others had trained themselves into unintended apathy ie. they had blunted their emotions in a quest to avoid being hurt which left them with wooden feelings. Some confused visualisation with fantasy and unwittingly travelled towards hallucination[50]. In any event, all were helped by correctly learning Stillness Meditation. However, it them took longer than someone without prior meditative experience as they needed to "unlearn" their unwelcome mental state.

Onflow of Stillness Meditation

Profound, Prolonged Reduction in Anxiety

A profound and prolonged reduction in the level of anxiety (see earlier) is a crucial element. There are two aspects:

---

48 Meares A (1968). Int J Clin Exp Hyp. 16(4):211-4. *This discussion regarding hypnosis without phenomena dates to before use of the term mental ataraxis.*
49 Meares A. A Better Life. 1989; Meares A. The Wealth Within.1978; Meares A (1977). Med J Aust 2(4):132-133.
50 Meares A. The Wealth Within. 1978.

- Duration of Meares' Stillness Meditation.
- The Onflow (outside of meditation practice).

These are outlined below.

Duration of Stillness Meditation

Whilst learning, Dr Meares' cancer patients meditated several times for short periods daily (ie. 2-4 x 10-15 min/day). After a couple of weeks or so the time was extended. In many instances, these patients attended Meares' meditation classes daily for a week or two.

Often, by the time they started with Meares they were weak from the cancer. Even the simple act of sitting on a chair during meditation practice was fatiguing. In a couple of weeks their strength improved. Also, the patient then had some experience of Stillness Meditation. At that point, the duration of Stillness Meditation was lengthened. Typically, the patient continued to use a chair or lay down on the floor, as the physical limits of age or illness made more difficult meditation postures unworkable[51].

Some meditated for 1-2 hours/day. Some meditated for several hours per day. The purpose of long duration is to help erase the aberrant physiological response. To wipe the slate clean, so that a better physiological response can replace it.

It should be realised that this is a distinct use of Stillness Meditation in regard to cancer (and certain similar diseases). For other applications 10-15 minute, 2-3 times per day is sufficient. However, regardless of the duration of Stillness Meditation, the Onflow is an important factor as well.

The Onflow

To meditate, say 1-2 hour a day, and then allow the stress of life to increase anxiety during the other 14 waking hours is ineffective. The effects of Stillness Meditation need to flow onward into all the waking hours of daily life. If the effects flow onward then, the cancer patient was no longer stressed by problems that they faced.

Meares' cancer patients spent hours in Stillness Meditation daily. But, more than that was needed for full effect. The effects of meditation must flow onward into the cancer patient's everyday life. Meares concluded that those who got the most from Stillness Meditation experienced a high Onflow. This Onflow is the continuance of the effects of Stillness Meditation in the alertness of everyday life. It is not due to the persistence of Stillness per se. It is a deep seated change in psychological reaction occurring in full alertness. In other words, a "new" normal waking state.

---

[51] *Meares' posture progression is in* Ainslie Meares on Meditation.

In its **early stages**, the Onflow is characterised by:
- calm of mind,
- coordinated ease of bodily movement, and
- a smooth appropriate response to stimuli ie. neither sluggishness nor over-reaction.

The Onflow is an important factor in maintaining a reduced level of anxiety. But, it does not stop there. Meares observed that it expands to enhance the psychological integration of the individual. The individual with **high Onflow** becomes:
- more philosophical,
- more understanding, with a sense of being part of all that is around them, and
- much more secure within (a greater sense of inner security as opposed to material security).

Meares[52] wrote: *"As far as his illness allows... the patient is still engaged in the realities of day-to-day living, but... becomes aware of experiencing a new dimension to his life... I have noticed also that still further change develops... He comes about his cancer [and] I lead him into this intense experience of Stillness Meditation, and he comes to experience life in a slightly different way... he becomes more interested in his changed experience of life than in his cancer. In this new orientation, the relief of his cancer becomes a side effect of the greater experience, a bonus that may eventuate"*

If I don't will the cancer to go,
what can I do?

You let it go,
You let the healing come
And the cancer responds.
It's as simple as that[53].

---

52 Meares A (1979) The Practitioner. 222(1327): 119-22.
53 Meares A. Cancer Another Way. 1977. pg103

Those who seek ease through meditation
Should remember well
The different kinds of meditation.
Those who concentrate their thoughts,
Or remain aware of breathing,
Or constantly repeat a mantra,
Or visualise,
Or meditate in real discomfort
Keep their mind alert,
And never achieve
That particular type of cerebral function
With the mind effortless and still.
In a state of complete tranquillity,
Which I believe to be so important[54].

---

54 Meares A. Let's Be At Ease. 1987. pg50.

6. Individuals & Outcomes

Meares' Cohort

A cohort is a group of individuals. Doctors use this term to describe a group sharing a common trait that is part of a clinical study observed over time.

Meares' cancer cohort. Meares' found that all those in his cohort who learnt Stillness Meditation got substantially reduced tension, anxiety, fear and pain. They experienced improved quality of life and were often able to reduce or abandon pain medication[55]. This was later on, after they had learnt Stillness Meditation.

In some cancer patients, cancer growth slows or it shrinks. Cancer doctors call this "regression". It is not to be confused with atavistic regression. Amongst those with lump shrinkage there were some whose cancer completely disappeared. This is described as a "remission". This strange term is used, as it is difficult to prove that every cancer cell down to the very last is gone. If the patient lives much longer than expected and dies of something unrelated to cancer then it is said that they had "remained in remission". Or, it was a permanent remission.

Some people, including some sad and hopeless cases, go into remission. When the doctors can find no reason for the disappearance of the cancer, it is called a "spontaneous" remission. It might be a surprise to learn that there are many reports of spontaneous remission[56], going back a long way, as far as the Egyptian Ebers Papyrus (1500BC). Meares' believed that the many cases of spontaneous remission were due to the same mechanisms operating in people who learnt Stillness Meditation (see earlier).

---

[55] *Only medical input permitted altering prescriptions to reduce dosages.*
[56] *Some reviews on spontaneous remission are listed:* Everson TC & Cole WH. Spontaneous regression of cancer. 1966; Boyd W. The spontaneous regression of cancer 1966. Challis GB & Stam HJ (1990) The spontaneous regression of cancer: a review of cases from 1900 to 1987. Acta Oncologica,29:545-50; Tadmor T (2019) Time to understand more about spontaneous regression of cancer. Acta Haematol 141:156-57; Niakan B (2019) Common factors among some reported cases of the spontaneous remission and regression of cancer. Int J Cancer Clin Res 6:112.

Benefits to be Expected

In 1980, Meares[57] reported, in an Australian medical journal, that new cancer patients taking up Stillness Meditation could expect:
- Less anxiety and less depression.
- Less discomfort and less pain.
- Better tolerance of the unpleasant side effects of chemotherapy and radiation.
- Improved quality of life.
- Death with dignity.

Some individuals in his cohort experienced one or more of the following benefits:
- Slowing of the rate of growth.
- Regression (shrinking) of the growth.

Overall, there was less chance of a recurrence of the cancer.

Group Results & Individual Cases

Injury, immune response and other factors vary for different cancers. Individuals with the same cancer will also vary.

A group of sick people can have a condition with the same label, yet there can be individual variability. There can be sub-categories that reflect different factors. Some sub-categories may be known to science. Other sub-categories may be unknown. This all influences individual outcomes.

No one may know which subcategory the client with cancer fits in and where they fit on the spectrum of individual variability. It is not known how the sick client relates to the group. A reliable prediction is that Stillness Meditation will provide the benefits mentioned above. However, the amount of help for a given individual is only known in hindsight. The extent of the benefit is only known later on. Benefit is expected. Extent known later on.

A client with cancer who wishes to learn Stillness Meditation already knows they have cancer. Stillness Meditation reduces anxiety and this improves mental wellbeing. Reduced anxiety relieves immune-suppression. This helps the immune system detect and kill the cancer cells. A profound and prolonged reduction in anxiety will result in substantial benefit over the fullness of time. Those who closely follow Meares' instructions and became skilled in Stillness Meditation will do better, closer to their own unique personal best outcome.

---

57 Meares A (1980). Aust Fam Physician. May 9(5):322-5.

© O Bruhn 2022

Combining Treatments

Introduction. Stillness Meditation teachers need to advise clients of any potential adverse interactions between Stillness Meditation and other medications or treatments[58]. The Stillness Meditation teacher provides general information (but not medical advice!).

Some people who learn Stillness Meditation experience slowing of growth or shrinkage of the lump. If the cancer client hopes to be one of them, they need to consider interactions between treatments. Treatments can be categorised by combined effect:[59]

- Independent ie. they have separate beneficial effects.
- Additive ie. both exert the same effect and this adds together.
- Antagonistic ie. the effects subtract from each other.

Often, treatments are independent or have an additive effect. The result is a positive benefit which is straight forward enough. In a few cases, treatments have an antagonistic effect and subtract one from the other.

The above principles are applied to common treatments below.

Surgery. By the time there is a lump the cancer may have spread. Cutting out and removing the lump makes it easier for the body to cope with any cells that have spread. The client may decide to learn Stillness Meditation and choose to have (sensible, non-heroic) surgery. General principles indicate that there should be a reasonable prospect of benefiting from both.

Medical immunotherapy. Medical immunotherapy refers to a range of treatments including those developed since Meares' time. Immunotherapy and Stillness Meditation both help by strengthening the immune response. General principles indicate that there should be a reasonable prospect of benefiting from both.

Radiation and chemotherapy. Radiation and cytotoxic drugs both kill cancer cells. They kill other cells including immune cells. This weakens the immune response. The beneficial effect of Stillness Meditation on the immune system are offset against damage from cell killing drugs and or radiation ie. an antagonistic effect.

Meares writes that:
- Some patients learning Stillness Meditation decided to avoid

---

[58] National Code of Conduct for health care workers. COAG Health Council 2015. Refer item 1(2)(h)... "*must have a sound understanding of any possible adverse interactions between the therapies and treatments being provided... and any other medications or treatments,... that he or she... should be aware that a client is taking... and advise the client of these interactions.*"

[59] *Other less common combined effects exist. They are beyond this discussion.*

radiation and chemotherapy. They hoped that their immune system would work better although more rogue cells would have to be removed by Stillness Meditation.
- Other patients opted for Stillness Meditation plus radiation and/or chemotherapy. They hoped that the radiation and/or drugs would kill a lot of cancer cells and that their immune system would rapidly recover. The next stage, being that Stillness Meditation, would help their immune system remove the remaining cancer cells.

Meares fully informed the patient regarding treatment(s) and the final decision was then entirely up to the patient.

Avoid Providing Medical Advice

Some medical doctors don't have the details about Meares' work. So, there is a need for generic information. The Stillness Meditation Teacher can't provide medical advice (unless they are a medical doctor, too). Teachers should take care to avoid crossing a line. If general information is not enough, then additional medical advice can be sought by the client, if desired.

Explanation But Not False Promises

"8(1) A health care worker must not claim or represent that (s)he is qualified, able or willing to cure cancer or... terminal illnesses.
8(2) A health care worker who claims to be able to treat or alleviate the symptoms of cancer or other terminal illnesses must be able to substantiate such claims."[60]

Regulatory agencies are concerned about fraudsters making false or misleading promises that are "scams" that empty the wallet but don't influence disease. Many jurisdictions make cancer and terminal diseases cases of special concern. Clearly, the officials in these agencies take a stance for good reasons. Making false promises is unhelpful, unethical and breaches that law. Providing accurate information to clients is a good thing. The point also needs to be made that making overly negative claims is unhelpful and just as unethical. In 1980, Meares' wrote: *"The greatest single obstacle to the cancer patient fulfilling his (or her) expectations from Stillness Meditation has been the active opposition of some family physicians and oncologists to this approach... a number of patients have become discouraged, and... have become quite confused and distressed in a way that has made effective Stillness Meditation, very much more difficult for them.*[61]*"*

---

60 National Code of Conduct for health care workers. COAG Health Council 2015.
61 Meares A (1980). Aust. Family Physician V9(6): 322-325.

Various ethical codes, including the medical code, state to the effect that the provider must "do no harm". Helping or no harm. Health practitioners are aware of the placebo and nocebo effects. They should not engage in words or actions that evoke the latter.

In 1977, Meares wrote: *"Doctors are human beings trained and conditioned in the science and art of medicine as it is understood at the time. Once trained and conditioned, it is hard to change. We ourselves know this from our experience of life. It is easy to advance new methods within the framework of the old. A new operation for cancer, and the surgeon will try it. New drugs are tried, even before they're fully tested. But with something different it is so very much harder to break with tradition and give it a trial."*

By 1983[62]: *"the problem is being resolved as doctors become more aware that therapeutic Stillness Meditation can be a viable alternative".*

In 2023, some 40 years later, more medical doctors are open to the use of Stillness Meditation to help cancer patients. However, some remain unaware of Meares' pioneering work.

Meares counselled that: *"logical understanding is necessary in order to give the patient a rationalisation for continuing with his meditative practice and, equally important, to give him some rational defence against the inevitable negative suggestions."*[63]

A **generic** explanation about how Stillness Meditation helps the cancer client will provide confidence. It will also help them to resist any inappropriate and negative suggestions made by others. The client also needs to consider what practical help and emotional support they can get from other people around them. General discussion may help them to identify sources of support.

A Full Time Client Commitment

Some people who have learnt Stillness Meditation have experienced lump shrinkage or remission. The cancer client hoping for this to occur must commit full time to Stillness Meditation. Several hours each day, 7 days a week. No days off. Enough time needs to be spent in Stillness Meditation to erase the dysfunctional reaction and allow a beneficial one to replace it. Yet, there is no forcing, or making it happen. In the experience of Stillness these things happen of their own volition. One creates the conditions rather than the outcome.

The human race became adapted to certain condition during our

---

62 Meares A (1983).Winthrop Impulse 22(6): 1-2.
63 Meares A (1979).The Practitioner. 222(1327): 119-22.

evolution. If we stray outside these conditions then adverse changes may occur. Creating the right conditions supports Stillness Meditation. For example, things like sufficient sleep. Insufficient sleep reduces healing.[64] Maintaining the Stillness Meditation support factors within the parameters' nature intended helps to support Stillness Meditation (see Ch. 15).

Conclusion

In conclusion:
- It is a general principle that clients be fully informed so that they can decide what is best for themselves (also Ch. 24).
- Meares' cohort results refer to outcomes for groups.
- Individual positions vary within that group.
- Individual outcomes are only known in hindsight.
- An individual's personal best Stillness Meditation outcome results from closely following Meares' Stillness Meditation instructions (including support factors).
- Stillness Meditation Teachers must avoid anything that:
  - resembles a false promise, or
  - might be mistaken for medical advice ie. only provide generic information.

The next chapter disentangles Meares' Onflow from some unrelated terms.

---

64 Xu X, Wang R, Sun Z, Wu R, Yan W et al (2019). Trehalose enhances bone fracture healing in a rat sleep deprivation model. Ann Transl Med.7(14):297.
Agness C, Tembo VP (2009). Factors that impact on sleep in intensive care patients, Intensive and Critical Care Nursing, V25(6):314-322. *Cites reviews of this topic.*

© O Bruhn 2022
7. Onflow & Other Terms

Introduction

From time to time, when discussing the Onflow of Stillness Meditation some people mention "going with the flow" or "being in the zone". This chapter describes the origin and meaning of these terms. It discusses how they relate to Meares' Onflow.

Go with the Flow

A Short History of Flow

Etymologists study the history and origin of words. They believe that "pleu[65]" is an ancient root of many words. For example, flow, flying, float, flee, fly, flea, flotsam, flood, pleura and plough (as in plough the earth). Perhaps, prehistoric creatures who were nearly human compared being alive with the magic motion of flying birds, flowing water, flowing stars and constellations in the sky. They were fascinated by swans and raptors. Yet, flowing water is to Earth what birds or stars are to the sky. In arid lands, water gives life.

The Greeks invented Stoicism a philosophy based on knowledge, living in harmony and indifference to the ups and downs of fortune, pleasure and pain. Zeno, the first Stoic, talked about "a good flow of life" and "living in alignment with nature"[66]. Others all the way to the Stoic Roman Emperor, Marcus Aurelius, wrote similar ideas[67]. An ancient widespread idea in Asian cultures is that of a person flowing like water in life or combat[68].

Shakespeare[69] wrote:
We at the height are ready to decline.
There is a tide in the affairs of men
Which, taken at the flood, leads on to fortune;

---

65 Watkins & Calvert (1985), "pleu-" in The American Heritage Dictionary of Indo-European Roots; Pokorny, Julius (1959) Indogermanisches etymologisches Wörterbuch [Indo-European Etymological Dictionary] (in German), vol 3:835–7; Rix, Helmut, Ed (2001); "*pleu̯-", in Lexikon der indogermanischen Verben [Lexicon of Indo-European Verbs] (in German), 2nd Ed, pp 487-8.
66 *Alignment may also be translated as agreement.*
67 Stoicism. Stanford Encyclopedia of Philosophy. Apr 10 2018.
plato.stanford.edu/entries/stoicism/
68 *Lao Tzu, the founder of Taoism recorded many quotes with the flow idea.*
69 Julius Caesar IV ii. 269–276. *Lines spoken by Brutus.*

> *Omitted, all the voyage of their life*
> *Is bound in shallows and in miseries.*
> *On such a full sea are we now afloat,*
> *And we must take the current when it serves,*
> *Or lose our ventures.*

The rhyming term "go with the flow" has been widely used since around 1920[70] and was very popular in the 1960s when the late psychologist Mihaly Csíkszentmihályi (sounds like: Cheek-sent-me-hi) was completing his PhD.

Csíkszentmihályi's Flow

Early in his career, Csíkszentmihályi studied artists, creative people, and then athletes. He concluded that they became engrossed in what they were doing: experiencing play rather than work. Later, he described "play" as flow. Flow is in the title of his 1974 grant report[71]. By 1988-1990, flow was used in various book titles[72]. After 1990[73], flow was added to the titles of some of Csíkszentmihályi's earlier works.

Csíkszentmihályi believed that his flow state was "related" to several other mental states. These include: Maslow's peak experience and, some meditation and religious states. His idea was that being engrossed in the task permitted passing into flow[74]. Managers and HR love the idea of focus resulting in higher productivity.

Nine components are said to be involved in achieving "flow": challenge-skill balance, merging of action and awareness, clarity of goals, immediate and unambiguous feedback, concentration on the task at hand, paradox of control, transformation of time, loss of self-consciousness, and "autotelic" experience.

"Autotelic" people find a task intrinsically rewarding. HR like the idea of a trait that involves enjoying work that others find miserable.

---

70 *Many sources say so with no actual verifiable references provided or identified.*
71 Csíkszentmihályi M (1974) FLOW studies of enjoyment. PHS Grant Report N RO1 HM 22883-02. N*ot sighted - it is only in a couple of overseas libraries.*
72 Csikszentmihalyi M & IS eds. Optimal Experience: Psychological studies of flow in consciousness. 1988. Csikszentmihalyi M. Flow: the psychology of optimal experience. 1990.
73Csíkszentmihályi M(1975) Play and intrinsic rewards. J Hum Psych 15(3):41-63 *(sighted). Flow is not in the original title but appears in later citations;*
Csíkszentmihályi M. Beyond Boredom and Anxiety: The Experience of Play in Work and Games.1975 *(sighted). This changes in the 2000 Ed to:* Beyond Boredom and Anxiety: Experiencing Flow in Work and Play.
74 Csikszentmihalyi M. Flow: The Psychology of Optimal Experience. 1990.

Meares' Onflow

Meares' idea of the onward flow of Stillness Meditation is straightforward. Simply put, the experience of Stillness Meditation results in an onward flow of calm and ease (see Ch. 5).

Onflow and Flow

Did Meares' pick up the word Onflow from Csíkszentmihályi's work? Did Csíkszentmihályi derive flow from Meares? Does it matter? Probably not. Except, to avoid confusing two distinct ideas.

Analogies comparing life and flowing water have existed since the time of primitive ancestors who could talk. "Going with the flow" was a popular term in the 1960s. Meares' first used the term Onflow in the mid1970s. One of Csíkszentmihályi' rare publications (unsighted) dates his use of "flow" to a similar time. It is not known if either knew of the other's work, let alone their specific terminology! One was a psychiatrist. The other a psychologist. They worked in distinct areas on different continents. Both Onflow and flow are separate words listed in dictionaries. It seems they each found a word to describe distinct concepts derived from their different approaches. The main point is to avoid mixing or confusing two distinct ideas.

Being in the Zone

Being in the zone (or groove) is sometimes used to describe being in Csíkszentmihályi's flow state.

The original "zone" was an item of clothing. It was the girdle worn by ancient Greek women at the hips. Astronomers keen on using Greek used this word to describe regions or areas in constellations and the night sky.

The term "zone" has been applied to team sports defense for a long time[75]. In late 1950s there was a popular TV program "The Twilight Zone" which had many seasons run over subsequent decades. This program and its actors also spread use of the word.

In the 1990s, an Ayurvedic practitioner wrote about physical training leading to "being in the zone", meaning excellent sports performance[76]. There was also an unrelated diet book by another author[77]. The sports and diet books both propagated wider use of "being in the zone".

---

75 *Various unreferenced sources claim the 1920s, however, no citation or rationale for that timeframe has been found.*
76 Douillard J. Body, Mind, and Sport. 1994
77 Sears B. The Zone Diet. 1995. *Mentioned for the its use of the word "zone".*

Being in the Groove

"Being in the groove" has a very simple history. It was derived from playing records on early phonographs and was sometimes shortened to a single word:- "groovy". When the sensor is in the groove of the rotating record it read the signal and converted it to music. Being in the groove creates harmony in the form of music. Before phonographs one had to be either wealthy and own a musical instrument or attend a community gathering to listen to others playing music. So, the phonograph enabled many people to listen by being in the groove whenever they wanted.

Conclusion

Using sayings about flow, zones and grooves can help communicate a vague idea about mental states. The reader should see that different people might assign different meanings to these terms. Erroneous understandings can be compounded. Better instruction can provide easier to read sign posts that highlight the path towards the experience of Stillness.

Whilst, a passing reference might be helpful, it is better to stick to Meares' term Onflow. This avoids the potential for misunderstanding albeit that some explanation of "Onflow" is also needed. Alternatively, the term being calm and at ease in daily living can be used, instead..

Meares' meditation involves relaxation, there is no task or focus per se. Relaxation is the opposite of trying or effort. Relaxation is effortless. The depth of Stillness involves letting go, letting it happen so it seems as if it happens almost by itself.

The Onflow of calm and ease occurs after Stillness Meditation. It does not involve focus but is effortless. One can be calm, relaxed and at ease whilst one is going about doing things.

Enough chasing rabbits down rabbit holes, or is that lepores flowing into grooved underground habitation zones? The next section returns to the topic of Stillness Meditation teaching. Fewer footnotes too!

S3. Meares' Medical Protocol

Note: This section distils Ainslie Meares protocol from his writings (refer S6 Bibliography). The Author's observations as a meditator in Meares' classes and the recollections of others are referenced by footnote.

8. Becoming a Stillness Meditation Teacher

"My own genuine ease of mind is the most important single factor in preparing the patient for meditation".[78] Ainslie Meares, 1982.

Know Stillness Well Yourself

After meeting selection criteria a person may attend university. They enrol, take subjects, pass tests and get their qualification. Next, they begin work, on-the-job learning and professional development.

So, we need to discuss what is needed to bring an individual to a point where they are able to implement Ainslie Meares' protocol. This is the individual's preparation to become a Stillness Meditation teacher. It involves more than reading a book. It is distinct from daily preparation to teach (Ch. 9) and ongoing development (Ch. 30).

To teach Meares' method one must become skilled at Stillness Meditation. One must let the effects of it flow onward through one's own life. One must learn to become calm in all that one does.

How long it takes depends on the starters block in relation to the finish point. Generally, people get a boost from about a dozen weekly Stillness Meditation classes[79]. This assumes that a person practices 15 minutes or so twice daily. To substantially develop the skill takes longer. Indeed, after 3 decades of practice, Meares wrote that he continued learning to meditate better and this further improved his own daily preparation.

Meares passed away unexpectedly before he set up a teacher training course. Today, in Australia, some (non-Meares) training courses are run over a weekend which seems far too short, even if the participants are very experienced meditators.

Meditation Association of Australia (MA) register training courses but also acknowledge that training as a meditation teacher may come from a number of sources with the onus on the applicant to ensure that the meditation teacher training they receive meets requirements for membership. Those without training at a MA registered course may be eligible for membership via recognition of prior learning. All applicant must be be able to verify that they have held a personal meditation practice for a minimum of 2 years.

So, it takes more than a couple of years to learn the basics and

---

78 Meares A (1982). Am J Clin Hyp 25(2/3):114-21
79 *Ainslie Meares comment to me. Observations of various people.*

train to be a Stillness Meditation teacher[80]. Some take up teacher training after practise of Stillness Meditation for a longer duration, as a long held goal or due to a change in direction.

The teacher needs to be able to "model" to clients, being a calm person in daily life. This does not require perfection but, to facilitate Mental Stillness in others you must know it well yourself.

Leadership

Over countless generation's evolution has built various psychological reactions into us. These reactions made it more likely that we survived. Any that reduced survival were rapidly bred out!

In primitive times, children looked up to parents and elders. When they grew up they looked up to leaders. These leaders were in a sense the parents of the tribe. Beneath the threshold of consciousness, they identified with parents and leaders, and learnt how to take on ("introject") the qualities they showed them.

They grew up with the others in the tribe and spent every day with the same group of individuals. Individuals and the tribe made survival decisions. Those who made wise choices were more likely to survive. For example, a robust, clever hunter tended to be a good provider and might come to be hunt leader. In time, someone who reminded us of the hunt leader, or past leaders who had joined the ancestors, might become the next leader. Food getting was important but, it was only one aspect of leadership.

In Chapter 3 we discussed how atavistic regression evolved. If there was no threat then the group relaxed into natural calm. This helped those in the group stay close together which offered protection. Those who wandered off by themselves were rapidly weeded out. Those mature individuals who were very calm influenced the rest of the group. It was subtle and harder to see than the hunter-warrior leader. Hunter-warrior leaders relied on prestige and authority. The calm leader had to rely upon a more passive approach. Sometimes, ambitious tribal members with little inner calm attempted to suggest calm to others who they hoped would accept their mimicry. This gambit usually failed as the others recognised it was fake. Today, this applies to some scammers and con people. It also applies to those who embark on meditation teaching without adequate preparation. Meares' wrote: *"we identify with a person who has a natural calm about him, we come to*

---

[80] Purely by way of analogy, to reach Reiki Master Teacher level recognised by the Aust. Reiki Connection requires 40+ hours of training over more than a year. The Master teachings are regarded as putting one on the path to mastery rather than completion. So the process becomes more like 1.5-2 years.

participate in his ease of mind... if... the hero displays ease of mind... we too are calm within ourselves. But if we identify with nervy restless characters, the quality of our life is reduced." [81]

This quote also reinforces the importance of facilitating mental Stillness in others after you know it well yourself.

Rapport in a Professional Setting

In modern times, we grow up, live, work and spend leisure with different individuals and groups. Many of us move and change jobs several times. Relationships are often just at one shared point eg. workmate. Very different from the old way within the tribe where we shared every day of our lives with the others.

In meditation teaching, rapport is *"the emotional state between student and teacher in a professional setting in which the student feels that he likes the teacher and can trust him and that this particular teacher can help him better than the others.*[82]

Meares' rapport[83] differs from the one sided calculating role assumed by psychoanalysts who let the patient's reactions deliberately transfer to them, so they can dissect them out in psychoanalysis.

Meares' rapport is a lot like the relationship individuals in the tribe had with the calm passive leader - it is the "same but different". The modern situation narrows it to the one shared point: *"a professional setting"*. The professional relationship excludes unrelated elements and acts to inhibit erotic feelings.

Meares[84] observes: *"the patient forms some opinion of us as soon as he sets his eyes on us... formal dress tells the patient that we expect a formal professional relationship..."*

The army, judiciary and clergy all have their work uniform. Modern TV doctors have the white coat and stethoscope. In Meares day, the standard attire donned before work by male medical specialists was a clean dark suit with tie. Whilst ensuring role appropriate formal dress, Meares styled long hair gave him a somewhat unconventional appearance. It helped youth identify with him. Adults saw him as an unusual doctor which fitted with teaching meditation as therapy, highly unusual back then.

Meares[85] points out that very formal dressing may make rapport

---

81 Meares A. The Hidden Powers of Leadership. 1978. p7.
82 Meares A. A Better Life. 1989. p40.
83 Meares A (1954) Lancet 264(6838):592-4; The medical interview, Ch.4. A System of Medical Hypnosis, Ch.12. Management of The anxious patient,Ch.17. Meares A. A Better Life. 1989. p40.
84 Meares A. The Medical Interview. 1957. p29
85 Meares A. The Mangaement of the Anxious Patient, p168-169

more difficult to attain with groups who dress very informally and are overawed by overly formal dress. Depending upon your client niche and setting this may also be a consideration (see later, Ch. 17). When working on drafting legislation and guidance and so on in a regulatory head office I found a suit and tie useful attire. But, when I spent time at the "coalface" sometimes at coal mines and other similar environments the dress code was very informal. I found I had to readjust it up again as I became more involved in Stillness Meditation.

There are many client niches, settings and occupational roles. In modern times, people of both sexes teach Stillness Meditation. They may wear a work uniform related to an existing work role and this makes a single prescriptive suit (or dress) unworkable. The modern "uniform" is clean, tidy and somewhat formal ("professional") in appearance, non-revealing with a minimum of scent and minimal jewellery. Not unlike dress for a business meeting. If needed, an easy to read watch will help keep a (relaxed!) eye on the time when teaching. The "uniform" sends subliminal clues that set the right formal tone for relationship as well as the use of "the space between" and soothing touch (see later).

From initial contact, the Stillness Meditation teacher builds rapport in the professional setting. Meares[86] writes: *Rapport achieved through unlimited trust... gives the patient the necessary security; he can then let himself go off guard and regress atavistically.* The modern non-medical teacher also continues to maintain rapport, shows the client their genuine calm and this extends later into the formal facilitation of Stillness Meditation.

The next chapter discusses Meares' recommendations for the ongoing daily preparation of Stillness Meditation teachers.

---

[86]Meares A. The Management of the Anxious Patient, p154

9. Daily Preparation to Teach

"I am still working on myself. Every morning. Still preparing myself. The hope is that I may come to do it (meditate) still better. So I speak to you as one of us, as it were" [87]

Dr Ainslie Meares, after 30+ years meditation teaching.

Meares' Daily Preparation

Morning Stillness Meditation

Every day, Meares' prepared himself to see his patients. In the early morning he would meditate for one quarter of an hour. In later years, this was often bare clad at dawn kneeling on concrete outside his apartment. Melbourne winter temperatures reach -3 C [27 F]). There is real effortlessness involved in transcending slight discomfort under these circumstances (also see Ch 30).

A Leisurely Walk

He would also go for a leisurely walk in a park located over the road from the rooms where he saw patients. The walk entrained the onward flow of the after-meditation calm and ease. Meares' believed that the genuine calm and ease of the teacher was **the single most important factor** in preparing patients for Stillness Meditation: *"This process has a very great effect on the patient, provided, of course, that the therapist [Stillness Meditation teacher] is genuinely and deeply at ease in himself"*[88].

Modern Daily Preparation

Daily preparation remains similar to Meares' preparation ie. practice of Stillness Meditation together with a leisurely walk and or a simple exercise "recharge" (ie. not a fatiguing workout). The recharge idea emphasises the cultivation of onflow.

The interfacing of physical activity, or any other activity for that matter, with Stillness Meditation is a big topic. It is explored further in Ch. 18 & 22.

Ch. 30 discusses ongoing development which is distinct from daily preparation.

---

87 Meares A. A Better Life. 1989.
88 Meares A (1982). Am J Clin Hyp 25(2/3):114-21

© O Bruhn 2022

10. Initial Contact

Finding Dr Meares

Dr Ainslie Meares' patients found him in various ways. Many did so by word of mouth. For example, from someone they knew who saw him. Or, "third" hand after someone they knew mentioned a third party who had seen him.

Over time, Dr Meares became well-known, appearing on radio, TV and eventually authoring 36 books. Some people have said that they felt they got to know him from his books and then went to see him.

Others who saw Dr Meares mention brief but leisurely conversations in public or at some event, and sometimes he provided contact details (via a card) that they used later to contact his rooms[89]. He also included his work address in most of his books and many articles he wrote and this was another avenue that enabled some people to contact him. Some people looked him up in the phone book (ie. this was before the internet).

Reception

Dr Meares' protocol started before the patient first saw him. The initial contact was usually by a phone call for an appointment. Meares' reception staff answered the phone in a natural unhurried way and were considerate to the new patient. This approach provided what Meares' described as subliminal cues as to what the patient might expect.

The reception staff usually recommended that the patient read one of Meares' books that outlined his approach to Stillness Meditation. There were several practical reasons for doing so.

First, reading one of his book(s) conveyed something of Meares' sensitivity and humanity so that the patient could more easily came to identify with and trust him.

Second, Meares' ideas while simple are subtle. Some reading meant the patient had a better understanding of what was involved before they saw him.

Third, reading beforehand reduced the need for explanation. Explanation increases logical thinking which prevents the slowing

---

[89] In 1984: *Ainslie Meares MD DPM, Consultant in meditation & hypnosis, 392 Albert St, E Melb . Ph:xx xxxx. Black ink on plain white card. Simple and elegant.*

and stilling of the mind.

You can see that Meares structured the entire process to commence a shift towards calm that started well before the actual commencement of Stillness Meditation.

First Arrival at Meares' Rooms

By first arrival we are talking about the time the patient entered Dr Ainslie Meares' reception or waiting room, before the interview with him occurred.

Meares put much thought into the design of his waiting room in terms of the physical environment as well as the interaction with his reception staff. The waiting room was quiet and comfortable. The reception staff spoke quietly and naturally to the new patient. The conversation proceeded in an unhurried, leisurely fashion.

Meares indicated that sometimes a new patient would arrive with relatives, and they would all be chattering away. However, typically the conversations slowed to gaps and then into a relaxed silence. Meares' writings emphasise that these things were not trivia. The details were important in providing the correct subliminal cues to set the scene. The patient who might be very tense and highly anxious could begin to relax and could later be bought to experience Stillness Meditation.

Meares' stressed that these important considerations helped to prepare the patient for that first session of Stillness Meditation. He believed that if these preparations were not adequate then the patient might abandon the idea of persisting with Stillness Meditation as being beyond his or her capacity. In other words, setting the scene for the first Stillness Meditation session helped to ease the person into it and the background of the success of that first session set the way for further success and progress at subsequent sessions.

11. Greeting & Preliminary Meeting

"When I am truly relaxed, there is a meeting of personalities, of his and mine and something happens. Sometimes it is all very still. He feels it; I feel it, and we are better for it. It is not all one-sided; when it works, I gain too." [90]

Greeting

In the previous chapter, we discussed how the patient first heard about Dr Ainslie Meares, made contact with his rooms and arrived at the rooms (usually) some days later. We left our hypothetical patient sitting in the reception\waiting area, having relaxed somewhat. We take up at the time the patient sighted Meares.

Dr Meares' always walked out to the reception area to greet his patients. He would offer to carry bags and show the person to his interview room. He would often do this by placing a hand on the shoulder or upper arm and steering the person along at a slow and leisurely pace. He might make some slow and easy remarks about some topic as he walked along. Sometimes, if appropriate, the short journey might be in a leisurely silence. Meares' approach was calming, reassuring and entirely consistent with the manners of his time (also see Ch. 16).

Meares' Preliminary Meeting

Seating & Meeting

In line with good manners at that time, he would help the patient take off their coat, take their bag & hat\umbrella and place these items out of the way. Often, this was on a hatstand on the way to his interview room. If he felt that an anxious patient might become more anxious if separated from their belongings he would help stow them safely in sight in his interview room.

After traversing several metres, Meares and patient arrived at his interview room. Casually, he would indicate the chair to sit upon and in a very relaxed unhurried manner, close the door. The patient felt it is as a signal of privacy and an announcement of the start of the next stage.

Then Meares would slowly move to his own chair, sit down, adjust himself to get comfortable and perhaps move some papers around on his desk. Meares said this whole sequence gave his

---

90 Meares A (1969). Med J Aust 1(16) 822-3

patient time to look at him and become familiar with him. He emphasised that it was as important for the patient to get to know him as it was for Meares to get to know them.

With the patient settled in, Meares would ask how he could help. This allowed the patient to tell him the reason(s) for the visit and what they hoped for. The details of the medical questions are beyond our scope here. However, the patient talked and asked him questions. Meares pondered them thoughtfully, each time with a pause. He introduced little gaps and pauses. Natural and relaxed pauses in which there was an absence of talk. Meares was very relaxed during these pauses. This resulted in the patient taking on some of his relaxation and it also added to the quite natural slowing down of the pace of conversation. The pauses gradually lengthened into natural silences. Again, this all contributed to preparing the patient for the Stillness of Meditation.

"*Bad things are catching-measles, anxiety and fear; so are good things- natural calm and ease... let us expose the patient to the latter.*"[91]

It must be emphasised that these pauses, gaps and silences must be sincere and completely natural. They must reflect genuine calm and ease. It is easy enough for an aggressive or tense person to deliberately pause but, if you think about it you will see that this has a completely different meaning. The faked pause may be felt as insincerity, tension, arrogance, or anger. Faking will sabotage by alerting the client. Hence, the need for adequate preparation by the teacher as discussed earlier.

Medical Exam

This section (S3 Meares Protocol) outlines Dr Meares complete medical protocol as it is recorded in his writings (with added observations of people who experienced it referenced by footnote). A Stillness Meditation teacher who is not a medical doctor must not attempt either medical examination (or medical treatment), as such. Adjustment is needed to ensure an effective NON-medical protocol is implemented (refer S4). But, before sensible adjustment can be contemplated or discussed, one must first understand Dr Meares' medical protocol.

Part of the medical protocol included a physical examination. The patient's doctor had provided a referral for the patient to see Meares with implied informed consent. At reception, the patient had filled further paperwork. In Meares' time, patients undertook a physical examination on an examination table. Consent was built in

---
[91] Meares A. (1969) Thoughts of an idle evening. Med J Aust 1(16) 822-3.

by requesting the patient to get onto the table to permit them to be examined which involved appropriate task related touch to measure blood pressure, heart rate, abdominal palpation and other tests that might be needed. Without derailing the text with detail, consent continued to be asked in simple ways. Raising the stethoscope was enough to indicate the patient needs to undo some buttons so the doctor may listen to the heart.

The examination needed to identify any physical signs or symptoms or confirm their absence. The relaxed approach Meares introduced earlier continued during the exam. This helped the patient to become used to Meares' close presence. The test procedures were adapted to simultaneously facilitate relaxation. He might lift the patients arm up a half inch or so and then let it drop or droop - encouraging the patient to feel the relaxation. The same with other tests. For example, repeating a knee extension reflex test and suggesting the patient relax. As they did so, encouraging them saying *"Relaxing, that's good"* or similar. Meares' approach allowed the patient to continue to relax. He found that patients would often let their eyes close with visible signs of physical relaxation present. The bigger picture is that all that had gone before was leading to further steps towards the experience of Stillness Meditation.

Stillness Meditation

On initial contact, Meares' reception had suggested that the patient read one of his books as a "quick start" to help learn Stillness Meditation. As mentioned earlier, this helped to reduce a need for explanation by Meares. Explanation tended to actively alert the patient which resulted in a step back from Stillness Meditation.

The next step was to "talk" the patient through the process of Stillness Meditation. Not explaining it but through the use of verbal prompts and cues as he sat in his chair or stood a distance away. A sufficient distance so that the patient did not feel encroached upon but close enough that they knew he was present to help them (ie. as a protective influence if they felt insecure or uncertain). "The space between" reflects many dimensions between teacher and client. It is discussed in a later chapter (see Ch. 13).

At the end of the session, Meares gently "woke up" his patient. There would follow some further explanation about the importance of relaxation and daily Stillness Meditation practice and that improvements were then inevitable which is the simple truth.

Initial contact to greeting, meeting and first meditation were small steps taken by Meares and his patient. In each step the patient calmed a little and made a move towards the Stillness of Meditation. There are also subliminal cues. There was a dim feeling that the next step, in the first group meditation class, was something they could achieve rather than abandoning their Stillness Meditation adventure.

Earlier, we discussed Meares' approach to the medical exam. At one point he, wrote a paper about how Dentist's might build relaxation of the patient into their dental examination:

"We do not tell the patient to relax, we communicate relaxation... we let him see that we are very relaxed in ourselves. Our speech becomes slower. Sentences give way to mere phrases. The rhythm of what we say follows the breathing of the patient... you as a dentist are in a favourable position to induce atavistic regression. You can communicate easily by touching the patient. The patient expects this, so it comes quite naturally. You put a bib around his neck. You adjust the headrest... You see that his arms are comfortable on the sides of the chair. You fiddle about with the headrest again... he senses the relaxation in your touch. Your hand slips down on his forehead, and... he closes his eyes and regression is further enhanced. When you remove your hand his eyes remain closed. As you do this, you make quiet grunts of satisfaction that all is well. These are made by breathing out just as the patient breathes out. In getting comfortable beside the patient you have occasion to move his arm just a little. Each of these contacts with the patient appears to have some useful purpose, but the main object of course is that communication. Your own ease, the way you touch him and your very closeness, allay the patient's anxiety and he is free to atavistically regress."[92]

---

[92] Meares A (1967) Annals Aust College Dent Surg 1:42-6.

12. Group Facilitation

Words are for logic;
grunts for things too deep for words;
touch for when it is deeper still;
and silence for when our inner being speaks.[93]

Elements in the Facilitation Sequence

Facilitation of Stillness is a simple organic holistic process. If we break it down into parts like in these chapters it sounds complicated, but it is not. A simplified overview may be helpful:
- The teachers' own calm and ease (Ch.8-9).
- Initial contact, greeting and meeting(Ch. 10-11).
- Greeting and seating.
- Verbal prompts.
- Presence.
- Wanted touch (Ch.13 & 19).
- The experience of calm community amongst the group.
- Waking up (Ch. 14).

This chapter (Ch. 12) discusses the sequence at the group meditation classes. The next chapter (Ch. 13) discusses aspects of the dynamics. To get the most out of Ch. 13. you will need to read this chapter first.

Greeting & Seating

The Stillness Meditation Room

Ainslie Meares' had large "wing backed" chairs placed in rows. All faced in one direction. He selected large leather Victorian wing backed chairs as they created a partial visual barrier between patients (see Ch. 20). The seated patients had privacy but, were aware that they are not alone and part of a group.

The number of chairs varied from 10 to 16. Meares' usually worked with a second facilitator who also provided wanted touch.

Greeting

At this point, the patient had found Dr Meares, attended the preliminary meeting and now attended again at the appointed time for a group session. Meares greeted each patient at the front door and took them to their seat in the Stillness Meditation room.

In keeping with formality and manners of the times, Meares

---
93 Meares A. (1969) Thoughts of an idle evening. Med J Aust 1(16) 822-3.

helped shift coats, umbrella and other items to a storage point. This helped to show care and his unhurried movement pattern showed his calm. It also removed clutter so he could easily move around the room during facilitation. A misstep might disturb the patients.

He encouraged patients to remove eyeglasses and to loosen any tight clothing (ie, so they could adopt a relaxed seated posture with hands in lap). They let their eyes close and began to relax.

Seating

Dr Meares' selected the most appropriate seat for each patient, steered them to it and helped them to be seated.

A shy **sensitive** type might be seated next to a wall or corner (on the edge and at the rear of the group). Over time, as the patient progressed, the seat changed so it was incrementally less isolated and then within the group. That shy patient learnt to experience a (platonic) interpersonal relationship with the facilitator(s) and this became a prototype for other interpersonal relationships. Meares mentions (if possible) it was preferable for patients to experience sessions with both male and female facilitators. A trained female facilitator assisted Meares in nearly all group classes.

Meares mentions that **aggressive** types were simply led into Stillness and this gave them an experience in passivity and calm. Repeated such experiences helped them to learn that no harm came from being more passive. They found that they had no need to be on guard and aggressive in their daily life.

An **arguing couple** came to see Dr Meares to save their relationship. He separated them at either end of his Stillness Meditation room. After several sessions he placed them closer and then next to each other. The gradual reduction in "the space between" (see later) helped them relearn to be a couple.

In modern times, manners may mean less formality. Some modern teachers greet clients and let them go to the Stillness Meditation room. The clients select a chair for themselves. A client who is sensitive and tense or has physical difficulties can, of course, still be accompanied to the room and helped to select a chair. In fact, an appropriate chair might be reserved (by sign) for a particular client. A couple similar to the arguing couple above might be advised to meditate well apart for the time being as things just work better that way.

Now, back to Meares' protocol. The patients are all seated and settling in. Meares withdrew to his office, meditated for a few minutes and then opened and shut his door (audible but not loud) on the way back in[94]. This signalled the next stage and a short time later the verbal prompts began.

Starting in non medical settings. Meares wrote that in a classroom the pupils might already be seated at their desks when meditation commenced. In a fitness gym, clients might be asked to assume a static posture (eg. laying down) and when they had done so, meditation could commence. The topic of starting in non-medical settings is also discussed in Ch. 20.

Verbal Prompts

"Please do not get the feeling that mental ataraxis is something complicated. It isn't... It is only the words that we have to use to describe it that make it seem complicated.[95]" It is: *"very simple indeed; like the thoughts and feelings of a child, so simple, so difficult, for adults to comprehend."*[96]

Stillness is a mental state, without thoughts per se, as the mind is resting. A book involves reading and words are the only vehicle of explanation. Prompts as Meares intended them are the simplest of ideas presented to patients. Each one suggests a feeling the patients then experience eg, starting with the legs *"The weight of your legs on the floor"* and the patients experience the heaviness and weight of the legs relaxing. Or later, *"Feel the face relax"*, and the patient's passive attention goes to the muscles of the face, and they relax them and feel them letting go. This is a very simple process. But to write or read about this simple process involves words, phrases (and sometimes a sentence). Each of them is a gentle reminder or prompt of feeling. Passive feeling rather than critical striving comprehension.

Ainslie Meares on Meditation contains a complete set of Meares' prompts dating from the late 1950s until the 1980s. They are quoted as written in the source. In some instances, transposition may be needed eg. "I" and "myself" transposed to "we" and "ourselves".

For this book we start with prompts from 1969[97]:
I just let myself go.
The weight of my legs on the floor.
I feel the weight of arms resting.
Feel myself sinking into the chair.
So relaxed.
I feel I am drifting.
Feel it in my face.

---

[94] Personal observation. *It seems Dr Meares used the door as a telegraph.*
[95] Meares A. The Wealth Within. 1978. p32
[96] Meares A. A Way of Doctoring. 1984. p18
[97] Meares A. Student Problems & a Guide to Study. 1969. p84.

Jaw muscles are relaxed.
Jaw muscles are so relaxed my lips part, and
my jaw sags with its natural weight.
My eyes close as I relax.
The muscles around my eyes,
I feel them relax.
Feel the muscles of my face as I relax.
Feel my forehead smooth out.
Feel the sides of the forehead relax

Our body is relaxed.
We are relaxed.
It is all through us.
Feel this.
Experience it.
It is natural.
You do not have to make yourself relax.
You do not have to do anything.
It is there
You just let it come.
It is quite effortless.
It feels good.
We enjoy it
We experience the feeling of the relaxation of our body;
we experience it in our mind.

Meares writes: *"The idea is to bring the patient to (atavistically) regress, so that he is no longer alert and critical. So I start by speaking in normal conversation, but I say nothing that requires any thought or answer on his part for this would keep him alert. I then come to speak more slowly, and the sentences become reduced to mere phrases. There are pauses between phrases and between words. The **cadence** of my speech corresponds to the rhythm of the patient's breathing*[98]*... it seems to give the patient some kind of feeling of unity with me; and with this there is a feeling of security, so he can let himself go off-guard."*[99] (underlining added)

Cadence. Sometimes, cadence helped by sighting the rising and falling of the shoulders and ribs cage, if clothing allows. Or, breathing may be sensed during touch to the shoulders and upper arms. If touch is applied without verbal prompts, there can be the gradual synchronisation of cadence of breathing of teacher with

---

98 *Cadence is yet another dimension of "the space between". See next Ch. 12.*
99 Meares A. (1967). Annals of Australian College of Dental Surgeons. 1:42-46.

meditator[100]. If the teacher is already breathing slowly then every 3-4th breath they exhale together with the meditator. Then, this slows to every second breathe as the meditator calms. Then even slower until it is 1:1 breath. Now, back to verbal prompts.

Going back to the 1969 set of prompts on the previous page, you might see that the length of some tended to build in unwanted oppurtunities for the patient to think. Some years later, Meares[101] provided some example short prompts for other teachers. They are quoted here without the gaps and pauses: *"Good; That's right."*... *"All resting; Feel the relaxation; Everything relaxed; Face relaxed; Eyes relaxed; Our whole self relaxed; In our face; In our mind; Our mind relaxed; Easy, natural, effortless; Body relaxed; Mind relaxed; Its all through us; The calm of it; Calm in our mind; More; Good; Really good."*

Shorter phrases and fewer words were Meares' way of providing simpler prompts. Simpler prompts promote a simpler response. An easy gentle slowing down in a prelude to Stillness.

These simple words were carefully chosen so that they were reassuring but did not result in critical thought in the patient. He used *"Good"* as an example of such a word. Another being *"Thats right"*. In both cases, they were spoken as a slow exhalation. The non-verbal phonation *"Ummm"* or *"Ahh" were* calming reassurance that he was close by. These were uttered as a slow exhalation. Over time, uttered like a sound of breath rather than a word.

His use of words continued to abbreviate and in mid1984[102] he ceased using words in his classes. In his writings around then, Meares accepted that teachers with less experience than himself would use more verbal prompts. A helpful bridge used for a few minutes. After the meditators have crossed the bridge, one lets go of the prompts. There is a lapse into silence as the non-verbal letting go of effortless relaxation quietly supervenes and the journey down the path into Stillness continues.

Meares explains that: *"When this has been continued for a few minutes the patients facial muscles are seen to relax. His jaw sags; the eyes are closed; and the expression becomes ironed out as it were. He is not asleep nor is he fully awake. He has in fact made this (atavistic) regression..."*[103]

Using the short prompts and phonation (*"Ummm"* or *"Ahh"*) of

---

100 Personal observation. *Footnoted for transparency.*
101 Meares A. A Better Life. 1989. p55, p68.
102 *I attended before and after the time in mid1984 he ceased using words. At the time, I wondered about the change and classes continued to go well.*
103 Meares A. (1967). Annals of Australian College of Dental Surgeons. 1:42-46.

his later approach, Meares emphasised use of sufficient prompts in the first two or three sessions: *"If we drone on too much we dull the students into a mental drowsiness. They are quite still and tranquil but drowsy... if at the first two or three sessions the students are somewhat dulled, it gives them a good start. They become accustomed to the unfamiliar state of Stillness. And they come to accept the experience we are offering them."* [104]

Therapeutic Touch

Background

Doctor, nurses, dentists, and body workers can't treat patients without touch. There can be no giving of comfort by health practitioners and carers without touch. Yet, helpful touch must be both wanted and appropriate. Informed consent is essential.

In Dr Meares' original medical protocol, patients were first seen in a medical interview that included a leisurely physical exam. The patient consents that the doctor listens to his heart, palpates his abdomen and elicits tendon reflexes etc. Obviously, thorough testing and accurate diagnosis are essential, however, an equally important purpose was to accustom the patient to relaxing, whilst Meares was nearby. This helped to build the circumstances needed for further communication by touch during class that aided relaxation.

This section describes Meares' use of touch in his meditation class. Touch **must** be adjusted for use by **non-medical** Stillness Meditation teachers in **modern times**. Sadly, touch can be fraught. The reader will need to carefully consider their own situation and weigh up the risks and benefits of the use of therapeutic touch. Also see Ch. 13, 19 & 24.

Therapeutic Touch & Atavistic Regression

Our race did not always have language and words. Distant ancestors made sounds of alarm, anger, contentment and so on. Then, some ancestors a bit closer to us learnt to use their minds intensely in thinking[105]. Periodically, they needed to temporarily regress and rest in the still mind state. Although, modern humans are more sophisticated, we are not that different. We also need regular time spent in Stillness.

The use of words alone in Stillness Meditation teaching is a limit. Words at the start, then gaps, pauses and soothing sounds. Finally, communication in silence by presence and\or by (wanted) touch to the shoulders-upper chest, back, arms and head.

---

104 Meares A. A Better Life. 1989. p25.
105 See Appendix 1, Still Mind Sound Body.

As Meares put it: *"In helping the patient.. I cannot communicate by logical use of words. If I use words to explain what I want, I alert the critical faculties... communication... is by verbalised phonation and by touch... similar... (to) mother and child."*[106]

"Touch says what words cannot say... "As we let our minds go still together, the process is greatly intensified by some degree of physical contact"[107]

This simple touch is pre-verbal and involves a simple feeling. To help to understand it, Meares' broke it down:

1. The touched one becomes aware of the touchers' state of mind eg. calm. The toucher knows if the touched one understands by the way touch is felt.
2. The touched one receives a message as a dim awareness (<u>not</u> a phrase). We can get a sense of it using words eg. *"I am calm, you can be calm, you are becoming calm... Our calm is his calm, our naturalness is his own naturalness."*[108]
3. Primitive processes can be awoken in the touched one's mind. Touch can increase calm and security. It must not alert. It is obvious, but must be said, that touch in meditation teaching must <u>never</u> communicate erotic love.

The General Sequence

Greet and seat. After the patient had been steered to the chair, Ainslie Meares sometimes rested the palms of his hands or a hand on top of the shoulders.

Armlift[109]. Earlier, it was mentioned that Meares gently lifted limbs during the medical exam and had already established this pattern of a small lift, flop and encouragement to relax.

Just after seating the patient, the patient's arm might be raised slightly and allowed to flop back into their lap. Meares gently gripped the wrist or forearm, lifted it a centimetre or so and let it drop. He said something like: *"Relaxing. That's good"* and then left the patient to greet and seat the next. On the way to greet the next patient, other shoulders were sometimes touched.

Up until mid 1984, after meditating for a short time, Meares formally commenced with verbal prompts which then passed into presence and touch. So, we take up the session at that point.

Rounds of touch. Patient were first touched on the shoulders which Meares' explained as allowing the hands to make gentle contact with the shoulders. The dynamics of touch are discussed in

---

106 Meares A (1980). Aust J Physio 26(1): 25-6.
107 Meares A (1969). Med J Aust 1(16) 822-3.
108 Meares A (1979). J Holistic Health 4:120-124.
109 *The arm lift formed part of Meares' protocol that he used sometimes.*

the next chapter (Ch. 13). Meares moved from one patient to another with one or perhaps two rounds of shoulder touch with each patient. Then in the next round, patients were touched upon the shoulders and then upon the head with both hands. There was no standardised formula for these rounds. Meares sensed "the space between" (see later) and did what was needed to help each patient.

As the rounds of touch commenced, almost imperceptibly, the group, including Meares himself, began to further relax. This developed quicker in some meditators than in others. It was essential that each patient was allowed to proceed at their individual rate. If the process were sped up beyond a patient's ability then they would be alerted and regression would slow or be temporarily lost.

Meares' continued this process of calming and wrote that as the Stillness deepened he had little contact with his immediate surroundings beyond a shared experience of the state experienced by the group. The group situation also had the *"the effect of the calm of the other meditating patients, and for a very anxious patient, the intensity and closeness is not so likely to be felt as threatening."*[110]

Silent Presence & Calm Community

The absence of "the space between" (see later) is silent presence and calm community. Then, the use of touch may cease.

Alternatively, a little more time may be spent with the ones in whom regression was slower to develop. When all was calm and very still, Meares' might remain standing so that the group was dimly aware of his protective influence. They sensed that he was watching over them.

Sometimes, Meares seated himself and meditated out in the front or within the group. There was a feeling amongst all of calm community yet, the group was dimly aware of him. The seat chosen may help to symbolise watching over the group. Or sometimes, it may be chosen to keep the facilitator closer to meditator(s) who are easily alerted from regression ie, so they feel the facilitator is nearby and can help them. Alternatively, the seated presence of the facilitator may give a dim sense of togetherness and sharing.

Closeness in a Shared Experience

Meares participated in the meditation and drifted in and out of the meditative state. In this way, Stillness Meditation was a shared experience. [NB contrasting with hypnosis where there is a gulf between patient and hypnotist].

Words make explaining the facilitation sequence lengthy and

---

110 Meares A (1979). J Holistic Health 4:120-124.

complicated when it is not. A repeat of the overview of the main elements may be helpful:

- The teachers' own calm and ease (Ch.8-9).
- Initial contact, greeting and meeting (Ch. 10-11).
- Greeting and seating.
- Verbal prompts.
- Presence.
- Wanted touch (Ch.13 & 19).
- The experience of calm community amongst the group.
- Waking up (Ch. 14).

Before we move to discuss waking up we need to discuss Meares' ideas on the dynamics of facilitation.

13. Bridging The Space Between

Bridging "The Space Between"

In oriental mysticism, loving and boxing (eastern martial arts) there are dynamic elements and changes that relate to "the space between". From mysticism and boxing there are metaphors involving a growing glimmer, crossing a bridge and unwanted separation from a mystic (or martial) moment by a pointing finger.

Ainslie Meares applied the oriental idea of "the space between" to Stillness Meditation teaching[111]. In oriental art, the gaps between individual subjects within a painting are as important as the objects drawn. Separation or closeness may be implied. There is significance in absence as well as in presence. The dynamic art of meditation teaching is only achieved by attention to "the space between".

The Auditory Space

The space between words is silence. Between thoughts it is Stillness. These things change as a session progresses. Then they change again after the session finishes and the mind returns to the normal waking state. Mental Stillness has been loosely referred to as "spaciousness", which may reflect a not so good attempt at translating "the space between" idea into English.[112] That is, the space or gaps between words (or thoughts).

From a slightly different angle, "the space between" starts with the meditators gathered within the Stillness Meditation room and verbal prompts commence. Then, verbal communication passes to silence and preverbal communication. The space between changes to one involving distance, closeness and touch.

The auditory space never completely disappears. The teacher moving about, breathing and so on continues to supply auditory cues below the meditators threshold of consciousness. In this way, the auditory space contributes to the physical space between.

The Physical Space

In the West, we say there is a space between us when the gap

---

111 Meares A (1967). Int J Clin Exp Hyp 15(4):156-9.
112 *"Spaciousness" is confusing. It draws attention to expansion. Effortless relaxation is a lessening and slowing. Spaciousness has no relation or relativeness unlike "the space between".*

sets us apart. Or, that we are distant from the person. We say we are close to someone when we feel things together with them. When we are emotionally close we say that we are united (or re-united, if we have been apart). Unison lacks separation. It lacks "the space between". Being in contact ranges from seeing, to proximity, to touch. Again, presence and distance or closeness are a dimension of the space between, or its lack.

Meares mentioned that many patients could be reassured by subtle movement towards them. However, patients were alerted if the approach was too close, too soon.

On the other hand, Meares' presence at greater distance increased the space between. The patient might feel that Meares was not close enough. Feeling abandoned or helpless as Meares' protective influence was to far away, out of range.

By gradually and slowly moving a bit closer, the right amount, this difficulty was overcome in even the most sensitive cases. The space between is neither too far apart nor too narrow.

A reduction in the space between by the teacher can nonverbally express something like *"I am here, I am helping you"*. It must not be too quick to avoid alerting. A slow speed is far different from a pushy forward lean. Ainslie Meares concluded that: *"skillful use of "the space between" brings a sense of harmony to... [Oriental] art. It can bring the same easy naturalness to... [Stillness Meditation] ...and the patient leaves us with a feeling of inner tranquility.*[113]

From Physical Space Between into Contact

The reader will need to carefully consider their own situation and weigh up the risks and benefits of the use of touch. Also see Ch. 12, 19 & 24.

If you recall times that you were a meditator in class you may remember that you were dimly aware of the teacher's presence before or as the touch arrived. There were various cues (of which you were largely unaware). You may have heard movement, detected shadows on your eyelids, felt the material on the chair shift slightly, the floor creaked or perhaps people in adjacent chairs shifted very slightly under touch or quietly exhaled or sighed in relaxation. Perhaps, the teacher exhaled (naturally) or you heard them moving towards you. Or, perhaps you felt the teacher superficially contact clothing fabric that shifted upon you slightly. There are very, very many cues at the threshold of consciousness. The net effect is an awareness of the teacher and touch shortly to arrive.

Meares wrote that he slowly moved to a place behind the patient.

---

113 Meares A (1967). Int J Clin Exp Hyp 15(4):156-9.

He paused so that a dim awareness of his approach dawned on the meditator. He mentions that the pause could be made while leaning on the back of the large wing backed chair which helped telegraph his presence. This may not be able to be replicated using some modern chairs. He also mentioned brief ever so light hand contact with clothing on the shoulder region before settling into the touch. The ideal timing resulted in the patient expecting the touch a little before it arrives. The main actions:

- a slow moving and relaxed approach,
- positioning behind the meditator,
- (perhaps leaning on the chair),
- the pause, and
- then the touch itself.

Those other visual and audible cues (see earlier) must not be contrived but spontaneously occur.

Meares shifted between meditators spending unhurried time with each one. A hand draped on the shoulder might gently drag along the shoulder as he moved on to the next. This helped communicate relaxation and a sense of moving on. The patient had a sense of *"now he is going but is still close by"*.

Stance and Reaching to Touch[114]

The teacher has to be able to reach the meditator to deliver touch. There are several factors:

- Meditator positioned at a convenient height by sitting on a chair. (NB excludes laying on floor and "exotic" postures).
- Floor free of clutter and tripping hazards.
- Enough space for teacher to move around and approach.
- Teacher assumes a comfortable standing posture. This includes weight on both feet placed hip width apart.

Depending on class size and so on, there may be 20-30 mins of static load on the shoulder by arms held out during touch. Although they are lowered as the teacher moves between meditators.

Shoulder and head touch may be done with the elbows bent. Sometimes, the elbows may be held close to the teacher's ribs. A short lever arm helps to reduce any fatigue in the teacher's shoulders. This is more likely to occur if the arms were held out straight and up at an angle (eg. a short teacher touching the head of a tall meditator on a high seat).

There is a need to stand further away from sensitive, tense people and the result may be straighter elbows. However, others can

---

[114] *This section is based on the author's ergonomic assessment.*

be approached more closely and this allows bent elbows that allow the shoulders to rest.

Further discussion regarding positioning of chairs and room layout is provided in Ch. 20. If chair design is suitable you may be able to place a hand on it to steady yourself, if needed.

Sites of Touch

Shoulders

Hands on shoulders. The palms of the hands make contact on the top of the shoulders. The finger drape and extend to the area just past the lower border of the collar bone (technically speaking this means fingertips are on the uppermost part of the chest). Those with short fingered small hands might not reach the chest.

Placement of the palm, near the first finger joints, rather than palm heel, on the top of the shoulders will place the finger tips higher so they may not reach the chest. It is also possible to place the palms on the top of the shoulder with thumbs forwards and the fingers draped onto the upper arm.

Meares' explains: *"the hand comes to rest on the shoulder and this is then felt. The fingers are allowed to drag on the clothing so that the patient is not taken by surprise by contact... initial contact with the fingertips, then the whole hand, as the wrist is allowed to relax in full flexion. Then comes the weight of the hand as it is released by relaxation of the muscles of the forearm. It is only when we are fully relaxed in ourselves that such a sequence is possible. It is this that brings the patient awareness of our own state of mind. The actual weight of the hand is followed by gentle pressure, and then a gradual upward movement."* [115]

Gentle lean on shoulders. Meares[116] sometimes leaned upon the shoulders with straight elbows. He very gently pushed down and then released (relaxed his elbows?) to take the load off the shoulders, as it were. The palm heel area touched the shoulders and then the lean happened. This involves a gentle lean using a small percentage of body weight. It is necessary to ensure it is not too heavy.

Dual outside gentle shoulder stroke (post-Meares).[117] One stands behind the seated meditator, and gently pulls or strokes down somewhat on the outside of both upper arms while allowing the palms to slide down the upper arms a short distance. This is

---

115 Meares A (1979). J Holistic Health 4:120-124.
116 *Personal observation.*
117 *Unique to FC. I feel obliged to catalogue it so it is not lost.*

done 2-4 times in rythmic moderately quick succession. Each outside shoulder <u>very gentle</u> pull results in the seated meditator experiencing a small natural reaction. First, the meditator is shifted slightly down into the chair, then their body reacts upwards and settles back into position. It is felt as being pulled down into the chair and then a short rise of a mere centimetre or so followed by an equally short shoulder "flop". There is a saying that a person who relaxes has a weight lifted from their shoulders. This technique, like the lean, adds a tiny weight to the shoulder and removes it.

To learn it, it needs to be practiced on a cooperative subject. It should feel enhancing of relaxation not repeated traction. If not practiced, it may be very alerting.

Head[118]

Touching the head may be undertaken after shoulder touch. The forehead and sides of the head near the temples are touched. Some care is needed as the face is out of sight when one is positioned behind the meditator. One way is that the hands are draped upon the shoulders. Then as the meditators calm deepens one slowly lifts the hands and places them upon the forehead and the sides of the forehead. The fingers are held gently together. The fingertips point forwards and the thumbs point towards the ceiling.

The fingers contact the forehead and then both hands move apart or stroke backwards till the palms are on the sides of the head around the temple area and above the ears. The little finger edge of the hands may be around the top of the ears.

Fine Tuning Touch

Unlike the black and white use of logic, touch involves feelings and errors can occur. These are dealt with by adjusting timing and delivery ie usually reducing closeness and lessening touch.

Some tips[119]:
- Too much touch, or touching too soon, can bring anxiety. This may mean delaying all touch. It may mean shoulder touch without head touch. The approach must be gradual, so the touched one lets themselves relax and is taken to deeper calm.
- Touch that makes the touched one wonder what is happening can bring anxiety.

---

[118] *Meares does not describe head touch in his writings although he mentions the Kings touch and laying on of hands (*Meares A (1954). Br J Med Hyp (Summer) pp. 1–4*). Touch to the forehead and sides of the head is a consistent feature disclosed by others who saw him.*

[119] *Tips mainly drawn from* Meares A (1979). J Holistic Health 4:120-124.

- Too light a touch tends to alert. Too heavy a touch may lead to a feeling that the teacher lacks sensitivity.
- Touching hands may be contaminated by empathy or sympathy. The wrist lift and flop is OK.

Also:[120]
- Keep hands and fingers well clear of the throat, eyes and ear canal. An alerting reaction has been bred into us to enable protection of vital functions like breathing and carotid arteries, vision, and hearing etc.
- Keep finger tips on or above the collarbone. Palms on top of the shoulders rather than the heel of the palm, if needed. Thumbs forward and fingers draped sideways down the arms may be used.
- Keep hands on the sides (ie. forehead and temples) rather than the top of the head as it feels more supportive.

Closing the Eyes – Only if Needed

A very tense person who is alert and looking about. Occasionally, a patient did not close their eyes after being seated. They remained tense and alert with eyes looking about in many directions. Meares approached at an angle, in line of sight (ie so they could see his reassuring approach). He then, slowly placed a very relaxed hand on the shoulder saying: *"Eyes closed and it comes to us better"*.[121]

A somewhat less tense person with eyes open gazing straight ahead. Meares writes: *"we let our fingers rest on their forehead. Then a few gentle stroking movements on the forehead. As they accustom themselves to this, we continue the movement but let our fingers slip down a little over the top of the eyes. Their eyes close. We let our finger remain there for a moment. Then let them slide on to the side of the face. Again, they rest there for a moment, and are then gently withdrawn. Our hands are on the shoulders again. And we quietly move off."* [122] This encouraged eyes to remain shut and reassured the meditator that Meares remained close by.

Sufficient Stillness Meditation practice will help reinforce the pattern of closing the eyes so it is well-established by time of first class attendance. Clearly, the emphasis is on ensuring the meditator is ready to change from 1:1 sessions to class rather than back up plan.

---

120 *Reasons provided are those of the author.*
121 Meares A. A Better Life. 1989. pg56
122 Meares A. A Better Life. 1989. pg56

14. Waking Up

Signal to Wake Up

In Dr Meares' protocol, group sessions went for 30 mins or so. Patients in the still mind state then needed to be returned to a state where relaxed natural thinking occurred (the normal waking state). So, the session was ended by waking up the patients. *"We must bring them out of it gently... In the manner that we ourselves are one of them coming out if it too"*[123]

A gentle waking. Too much volume will alert. Too little volume, too few words or little time in resting may prevent complete counter regression (see later). In 1984,[124], Meares quietly uttered "M*mmhhhh*". [pause] Then again, a bit louder "M*mmhhh*". [pause]. The third time in normal voice clearly heard by all "M*mmhhh*". [pause]. Then, incisively *"Good"* [pause] *"That's good"* (or *"That was good")* [pause] *"Just let your eyes open now"* [short pause] *Rest quietly for a moment"*. He left for a few minutes opening and shutting his office door which also announced his return[125].

The words can vary within limits. Two example sequences:
1. M*mmhhh. Good. Good. That's good. Just let... etc.*
2. M*mmhhh. Mmmhhh. Good. That's good. Just let... etc.*

If *"Mmmhhhs"* are difficult then perhaps *"tttTTThat's good"* instead.

Goodbye Backup Check

Meares then attended to each patient, one at a time. He retrieved umbrellas and any other chattels and offered to help put on coats etc. Then, he walked each patient to the front door. He checked (again) that they had undergone complete counter regression and undertook any "debrief" needed on the door step. This was a short distance to a busy street and the buzz of traffic prevented Meares and the patient being overheard by those inside as well as anyone outside who happened to be walking by.

Incomplete Waking

Just as it takes time for the whole group to regress, it took time

---

123 Meares A. A Better Life. 1989. p60.
124 Personal observation. *The first Mmmhhh was so quiet I was sometimes unsure if there were always 2 or 3.*
125 Personal observation. *The door firmly closing telegraphed his movements.*

for all patients to make the counter-regression back to the normal waking state. Some patients made it very quickly. A few made it far more slowly. Meares points out that they must not be prematurely "discharged" in a drowsy state ie. unfit to cross roads, drive etc.

After waking and resting Meares checked each individually during the walk and at the door so he was sure that they were fit to leave. Any that were drowsy had to wait until it was clear that they had regained normal alertness. He also mentions providing a cup of tea for the unusual patient whose drowsiness persisted for longer.

Order of Discharge

Patients who regressed quickly were checked and seen to the door first. This meant that the ones who were drowsy had more time to rest before being checked. If a patient was drowsy but unsettled (as sometimes occurred) then they were seen more promptly, taken to one side, reassured and either discharged or kept to rest further.

Motivational talk after wake up

Meares sometimes taught groups consisting of members of the general public. He signalled them, in the usual way, to wake up. After letting them rest for a couple of minutes, he talked incisively for 10 minutes or so on the value of reducing anxiety by Stillness Meditation, encouragement to practice and to return for the next session. Then, he moved to the door for individual goodbye checks.

Feedback & Reassurance

The check that counter regression has occurred, also provided an opportunity to respond to any questions and provide constructive feedback. Those who were unsettled or experienced a slow counter-regression and felt drowsy were reassured. Explanation was provided regarding variation in waking and the need to sit still and rest till they had woken up properly.

Meares notes that on arrival some nervous patients were unable to disclose something to him then. After the session they were able to disclose it. Selecting a suitable location for both goodbye check and any potential disclosures is important.

© O Bruhn 2022

15. Separate From Stillness Meditation

Introduction
Previous chapters make it clear that Ainslie Meares deliberately restricted the elements inside the Stillness Meditation room to those that were essential to facilitate Stillness. Other elements were kept separate. They are outlined in this chapter.

Mundane Matters
Meares kept mundane matters like administration, fees and so on separate from his protocol by allocating this to his reception staff. This meant that the patients were unconcerned about such things when they were with Meares. It led to a sense that Meares' only purpose was to help them.

In lean modern times, the teacher may not have the luxury of reception staff. Practical measures can still be taken to keep mundane matters separate in space or time. Dealing with such things separately from Stillness Meditation, having a separate admin area to discuss such matters, when needed.

In this book, Meares protocol has been kept apart from mundane matters in separate sections (ie, S3 and S5).

Explanation
Initially, reception suggested the patient read up on meditation from one of Meares' books. When Meares saw the patient there was minimal explanation while Meares was calming them. Next, direct experience of Stillness Meditation reduced the need for explanation. Then, class followed. Ch. 20 further discusses communication outside of Stillness Meditation.

Practice Outside of Class
Daily practice at home is intrinsically separate from class. It was not practical to teach some elements in class. Some people practised at home identical to class. Others gradually adopted these elements (outlined below) into their daily practice.

Meditation Posture Progression

It was impractical to use the progression in class:
- A range of postures would reduce group coherence.
- Some postures, like laying on the floor, make it difficult to touch the head and shoulders of meditators.
- meditators on the floor would be alerted by concern of being stepped upon as the teacher approached.
- Slip, trip and fall hazards might be created for the teacher.

Meares recommended a Stillness Meditation posture progression[126] for practice at home by those whose health permitted it. Meares mentioned his posture progression in conversations with patients and wrote it down so his readers could read about it.[127]

Making the Stillness More General

Experiencing Stillness in the chair was first, then the posture progression. The next step was to add distracting stimuli[128], thus making the Stillness more general. Introducing stimuli into class posed problems. First, some can't be transported. Second, the meditators skill varied. Too much distracting stimulus would alert some and make them tense up.

Anyway, Meares' mentioned ways of making the Stillness more general to patients and his readers read about it[129]. Also see Ch. 30.

Learning to Live Calm

The Onflow occurs in daily living outside of Stillness Meditation.

Supplements

Meares' "main dish" was Stillness Meditation and learning to be calm and at ease in daily life. Supplements include Meditation Support Factors and his poetry. Supplements were spices, or side dishes, that you can choose to add.

Experential learning[130]. Experiential learning can add to the meditators' move towards a better life. Sensitivity and social anxiety are used here as an example.

Evolution dictates that fineness of perception varies within groups of primitives. In the old way, ancestors hunted and gathered.

---

126 Discussed in Relief Without Drugs Ch.pp 68-71; The Wealth Within Ch.5; Life Without Stress Ch.8; A Better Life Ch.117-121 and many journal articles. It is also in <u>Ainslie Meares on Meditation.</u>
127 Personal observation. *Most other people who saw Meares recall this too.*
128 Discussed in The Wealth Within Ch.7; Life Without Stress Ch.8; A Better Life Ch. 5 & 11 and many journal articles.. It is also in <u>Ainslie Meares on Meditation.</u>
129 Personal observation. *Most other people who saw Meares recall this too.*
130 For example,The Wealth Within, Ch 9-13.

The fight flight reaction helped them to kill food, predators and enemies or to run away. The most sensitive discerned subtle signals and this allowed alerting to spread more rapidly with a quicker group response. This contributed to survival and having off spring. Finer perception is also involved in our ongoing socio-technical evolution. Meares believed that sensitivity was a gift that we should learn to use so we experienced things to the full that did not damage our inner self. Social anxiety is often associated with sensitivity. The help provided by Stillness Meditation and Onflow can be supplemented by practice socialising in easy situations without consequences. Hence, a person interested in, for example, collecting might join a club with others having that interest. Conversation is helped by having something in common and mistakes don't matter unlike a job interview or a date.

Meditation Support Factors. During our evolution we lived within the limits to which our physiology became accustomed. A gap between our way of life and those limits influences health when the human organism can't restore balance. To get the best results from Stillness Meditation we need to maintain such "Support Factors" within limits (eg. get sufficient sleep)[131].

Meares' mentioned the above supplements in passing to patients and his readers read about them in his books. He sometimes referred people to one of his books, mentioning they were readily accessible via a nearby bookshop located down the road. <u>A Key to the Books of Ainslie Meares</u> was written to help identify which of Meares' books might best meet your interest and is a better guide than guessing contents by title. The supplements are also catalogued in <u>Still Mind Sound Body</u>.

Poetry. Meares wrote poetry, 10 books of it, to help people learn Stillness Meditation. Of course, the poems were to be read outside of Stillness Meditation! <u>Ainslie Meares on Meditation</u> includes 33+ sample poems. <u>A Key to the Books of Ainslie Meares</u> has first line indexes of all of his poetry books for those who want to choose one that way. Or you might just get one his poetry books and dip into it.

Do read some of Meares' poems, if you have not done so. That puts you in a better position to mention them to clients. I go through phases of reading Meares' poetry books myself and remain surprised by the glimpses of Stillness they continue to evoke.

In S3 Meares' protocol started with meeting the new patient through to the "goodbye check" at end of class. This chapter has discussed how Meares' system extended outside the classroom. Yet, there are gaps. These are tackled in the next section (S4) and tips are

---

131 For example refer - Life Without Stress Ch. 5.

provided for the readers consideration.

S4. A Modern Non-Medical Protocol

Authors Note: This section (S4.) adjusts Meares' protocol and provides tips derived in part using health, ergonomics, consulting and training methodologies. The principles underlying Meares' work remain at the core of Section 4.

16. Same But Different

Occupational Role

Dr Ainslie Meares' protocol was a medical protocol. Today's Stillness Meditation teacher can't follow a medical protocol with a physical examination unless they are a doctor or "body worker" (eg. physiotherapist etc). Modern medical and body workers must touch in order to treat. They have an opportunity to follow Meares' medical protocol using appropriate touch within the context of their role.

The approach a physiotherapist, school teacher or a person with another occupation uses to teach Meares' Stillness Meditation will differ (within limits). Even the approach a school teacher might use to teach Stillness Meditation to pupils in class may differ from a different group in a different setting. The principles remain the same, however, there will be variations within limits. In short, a modern teaching approach must be the "same but different".

Interfacing with other methods – is discussed in Ch. 22.

Manners & Culture Change Over Time

Prior to the late 1950s, doctors offered a cigarette to patients as a friendly gesture that was good manners. Today, a doctor offering a patient a cigarette would make the patient anxious. They would avoid that doctor and might even report them to the Medical Board.

Meares' protocol and writings date from the mid 1950s to 1986. Manners and culture have changed since those times. Six decades later an effective approach needs to be suited to the culture and manners of current times. It must be the "same but different".

Modern Audience & Niche

The nature of the audience influences the approach too. Meares' taught patients in his medical clinic. Most modern teachers teach Stillness Meditation to clients in a non-medical setting. There are several categories of audience not limited to children, older students, adults, middle to silver years, end of life, athletes and other groups. Niches, audiences, settings etc. are discussed in Ch. 17. The point to be made here is that all learn Stillness Meditation but, the approach will be "same but different".

Individual Teachers

The author has been fortunate in having been taught by Ainslie Meares, MD and to have participated in classes led by a couple of dozen Stillness Meditation Teachers.

There is an element of individuality to teaching Meares' method. The same core elements are embedded but, there can be some variability in approach within certain limits.

Meares indicated that the verbal aspects of facilitating Stillness Meditation might be a bit more emphasised by those with less experience teaching. Some teachers use fairly similar prompts. Some weave a different "script" each time. Some use sound of voice in a relative simple way. Others are more lullaby like in resemblance.

All cease verbal prompts, as the session shifts into silence. The use of the space between and touch also varies. In all cases, it involves wanted appropriate touch after prior informed consent. The variation in touch is easily recognised via direct experience with different teachers. In all cases, touch helps the meditator to pass deeper into Stillness. Again, variation is within limits: "same but different".

In some instances, clients request that touch is withheld. Some occupational roles may be subject to policy that may limit appropriate wanted touch. Some teachers decide that touch is fraught and use "the space between" without the direct contact touch – hands may reach out and hover a few inches above the body.

In relation to touch, medical doctors and body workers have an opportunity to closely follow Meares protocol, adjusted in line with modern good medical (and body worker) standards of practice.

It should be clear that modern teachers appropriately adjust Meares protocol and this leads the meditators into Stillness. From the meditator's perspective, the protocol is not identical but is "same but different".

In *A Better Life,* Meares outlines an approach particularly suited to School teaching.

In the Holistic Health[132] article he recounts the use of atavistic touch used in both seated groups and one to one with patient laying down. In recent times, I have visited other meditative touch therapy systems. I can verify the effectiveness of the Holistic Health article approach and related concepts. The details will need to wait until this book is revised in due course.

---

132 Meares A (1979). J Holistic Health 4:120-124.

17. Helping Clients Find You

Finding Clients

If clients and niche already exist then, Stillness Meditation teaching may be simply added to an existing service. It is a matter of fitting it into class or clinic (see Ch. 16 & 22).

Others are starting from scratch. Their niche depends upon lived experience, audience background and special interest(s).

Niche Audiences

Meares' niche was as a medical specialist seeing patients in his clinic. Life cycle categories may help you identify your niche:
- Children - learning relaxation as a lifetime habit. Inside or outside the school classroom.
- Older pupils and young adults– reduction of anxiety, help with study, relationships and family.
- Middle to silver years - mysticism, meaning and health.
- End of life - to reduce anxiety, reduce pain, dignity in death.

Below is another generic set of categories:
- Sick people seeking therapy to reduce anxiety, better coping with pain, help with psychosomatic conditions, the hope of healing, dignity in death if facing the reaper. etc.
- Those seeking optimal mind body health and wellness.
- Athletes seeking to improve recovery in order to improve performance (as distinct from health).
- People seeking an enhanced ability for spiritual experience or anxiety reduction compatible with religious life[133].
- Non-religious people (eg. atheists) seeking science based anxiety reduction free of religious influence.
- Others eg. workplace groups, sensation seekers etc.

Your niche might be one or more of the categories on this list. Don't be blinkered. Your niche might be a variant not specified above.

Settings

A setting relates to niche audience, venue and location:

---

[133] *Meares' wrote that mysticism should be deferred until middle age. Teenagers and young adults can catapult themselves into psychosis by seeking mystic experience in meditation. Screening at registration and anxiety reduction by Stillness Meditation for 10-15 minutes twice daily substantially reduces the risk.*

- School classroom or hall.
- Gym or sports facility.
- At home.
- Dedicated venue.
- Leased or rented room or hall.
- Incursion to provided venue such as a workplace.
- Group excursion to venue provided by teacher or client.

One of more settings might be used. Starting out in one setting and changing to another later on might also be relevant. Considering settings may also help clarify niche audience.

Location is built into a physical venue. Ideally, the location is near homes or workplaces of enormous numbers of potential clients. Also, ample parking (low or no cost), public transport, taxi and bike paths nearby. The maximum distance or time clients are prepared to travel sets the size of your geographic "catchment area". Teacher travel time is also a further consideration.

Helping Clients to Find You

Clients Find "Problem(s)"

Ergonomists have observed that users find "problems" inside social systems as discrete patterns. The problem can be an element in the pattern or an absence (ie. that makes a pattern too)[134].

For example, some people find "trouble" stresses them. They liken "trouble" to a harmful substance. Each repeated dose causes inevitable emotional damage. This may frame solutions like drugs (medical or illegal) or lifestyle restriction. Of course, stress only occurs when people don't cope. Stillness Meditation reduces anxiety due to less than optimal coping. Learning calm and ease in daily life improves coping so people respond less to "troubles".

This is just one example. There are as many found "problems" as there are niche audiences and many within a single niche audience. People only see outside their "problem" frame with difficulty. Understanding their found "problem", can help to educate them so the effective solution is more conspicuous and readily mental accessible. In the "trouble" example, reframing it as better coping. Knowing will help motivate doing ie learning Stillness Meditation.

Systems That Help Clients Find You

You need to to reach out to your potential clients to help them find you. Some ways to do so:
- First and best are spontaneous referrals from:

---

134 Sims D (1979). A framework for understanding the definition and formulation of problems in teams. Human Relations 32(11): 909–921.

© O Bruhn 2022

- - Clients telling others about Stillness Meditation and new found inner calm are very helpful.
  - Allies (individuals or organisations) in parallel or related roles who mention your activities to their clients.
- Website(s) including search engine optimisation.
- Facebook & social media. What goes up on the internet stays up. Avoid dual relationships (see Ch. 25).
- A brochure and "calling" card will help clients (who find them) to remember and find you later.
  - Costing of card and flyer will influence distribution.
  - Flyers should also be in digital format to be downloaded from your website or sent as an email attachment.
  - Cards printed in batches and stock renewed when numbers reduce below some set point.
  - Card details should be in your email signature. Each email you send is a potential "calling" card.
- Mail:
  - Letter drop into mail boxes near a teaching location. Distribution limited by distance and time involved in walking. Response rate may be 0-5 per 100 flyers "dropped". 500 flyers might generate 5 clients.
  - Snail mail. Costly. Needs to be highly selective.
  - Email lists. Be sure to allow "unsubscription" to comply with Privacy law (S5) and courtesy. From time to time, someone will want no further information. Prompt removal from lists may even create good will if your calm, timely response is mentioned by them to others.
- Flyer's pinned up in shops, supermarkets and shopping centres etc. (many have notice boards or an area set aside).
- Other health providers may allow brochures or cards placed in their clinic. "Referrals" require the provider (or staff) to meet due diligence. You will need to provide support information to them (bio, quals, experience etc).
- Placement of your contact details on supportive websites.
- Writing articles, blogs and so on (with embedded details).
- Giving interviews and talks ie. digital or face to face. Venue provided by you or others involved.
- Involvement in industry, professional or other associations. Listings as (teaching) member and services offered.
- Phone follow up of contacts identified during the above activities. Having found you some may become clients. If not they may have useful ideas or further contacts.

- Remember not to be blinkered by this chapter. Lists are a great aid but can create a square. Think outside the square.

Further considerations regarding the above approaches:
- Approaches that focus on your potential client group\niche are better than a shotgun that scatters in all directions. But, too narrow might exclude some potential clients.
- Consider cost, time, and response rate.
- Clients vary in communications preferences. Face to face, phone, digital, paper are all needed. Your niche audience may have a distinct preference or preferences.
- There is risk in not having a website, brochure and calling card as some clients read the absence as reduced reputation, prestige and organisational stability.
- Include website, email etc. on everything.
- "Claims made" must be accurate and easily understood. Testimonials must only be used after careful checks. At start 2023, AHPRA registered providers were prohibited from using testimonials. See Ch. 23 & 25.
- Take enquires\enrolments in chronological order and remember a waiting list, if needed (happy days!).
- Evaluate outcomes to help improve your next approach so even more clients find you:
  - Did the message reach the people to whom it was sent?
  - Did they understand it?
  - Was the message sent to the right people? (Or, were some "misclassified" as clients A few misclassifications are probably OK, many is likely to be a problem.)
  - Was the response rate high? Mail drops often involve 1-10%. Costly options need a high response rate. Many (non-meditation) surveys consider 60-70% a high response rate (ie. 30-40% non reply). (Non meditation) consultants anticipate a lower rate eg. 1 in 3-5.
  - How else can the next approach be improved?

Consider writing down your niche, setting, and systems for helping clients to find you to clarify your own thinking. That gives you a first version of a plan to build upon. The plan can be fine tuned via further information including outcome evaluations.

© O Bruhn 2022

18. Greet, Meet & Facilitate

Communication Outside Meditation

Meares' protocol (S3), emphasised rapport and the need to keep explanation separate from Stillness Meditation (eg. Ch. 8-14). Meares strongly emphasised this in all his writings, yet it is not the whole story of communication with clients.

About 10% of adults can't read. They keep it a secret, but are truthfully adamant that talking is the only option. Some others who saw Ainslie Meares did so due to curiosity about "meditation" or at the behest of relatives. They tended not to read his books.

Rebellious teenagers taken to see Meares by their parents did not read books given to them by parents. Literate teenagers and adult wanting help always read Meares' books before seeing him.

It should be clear that Meares sometimes provided explanation prior to the initial Stillness Meditation session. He also had to explain how Stillness Meditation differed from other types.

The many models of training adults involve: gain interest & attention, instruct, practice and give feedback.[135]

Meares avoided the word "instruct". It sounds like teachers making pupils exert effort. Instead, explannation is offered to clients. This fits in better with the passive approach to rapport.

Meares writes of 3 components used outside of the actual Stillness Meditation session. **Explanation** concerns logic. Logic is often insufficient to motivate. Some people drink alcohol, take drugs or drive at breakneck speed. Logic makes clear the risks yet, they may continue to do so. Clearly, there is an emotional component to **Motivation**. **Rapport** is pure emotion without a logical component. Much of Meares' protocol is concerned with fostering rapport. Calm grows from trust and liking in the context of a formal teacher-client relationship (see Ch. 8).

In summary:
- **Explanation** involves pure logic.
- **Motivation** is a mixture of logic and emotion.
- **Rapport** involves pure emotion.

---

[135] Bruhn O (1990). Development, delivery and evaluation of a heat stress training program for an Inspectorate. Thesis for Grad Diploma Ergonomics. La Trobe University;

It is better if the client has already read a book. One way or another one communicates **what to do, what not do**, and **what to expect**. Once the client(s) begins to meditate, communication has already transitioned to rapport. This avoids rousing the logic faculties that will alert the client. Rapport allows communication of calm that helps the client's mind to settle down and still.

Experience reduces the need for explanation. The experience of calm helps reduce the need for explanation. Mental relaxation into calm, or even tranquillity, is a motivating experience. Understanding how anxiety reduction via Stillness Meditation links to your niche audience will also help your communication (also see example 1, over page). In your niche some clients may have psychosomatic conditions. They will feel calmed by Stillness Meditation but, also need to appreciate that daily practice for several weeks or so is needed until symptoms begin to reduce (then daily practice going forwards!). Cancer was discussed earlier (Ch. 5-6).

Some communication process variants

Scattered through his writings, Meares provides examples of "same but different". These are briefly outlined below.

Client Has Just Met Teacher. There will be a need for introductions, background etc. so that the client(or group) gets to know the teacher. Such interactions, of necessity, contain explanation about Stillness Meditation near the start. If a Stillness Meditative experience is included then there will be a need to shift the balance from explanation into rapport with slowing and quieting. See later, refer generic examples 2&3.

Experienced Clients. Stillness Meditation can commence with relatively little communication as soon as experienced clients arrive. In one approach the session finishes and the normal counter regression process is followed.

Motivational talk as the group or class wakes up. The class is woken as usual with a rest for a couple of minutes as the teacher deems appropriate. Then the teacher provides 10 minutes or so of explanation and motivation. This provides enough time and stimulation to help to ensure counter regression. It is backed up by the usual "goodbye" counter regression check. The talk might be about topics such as: the benefits of relaxation, daily practice and further benefits of attending future meditation class.

Discussion after counter regression. In a slightly different approach, after counter regression has occurred, the calm community of the group sets the scene for constructive discussion of Stillness Meditation related matters. The teacher provides explanation and motivation as needed. This process tends to requires more time than the others.

Motivational suggestion for practice outside of class.
The meditation "posture progression" and stimuli to "make the Stillness more general" are undertaken in daily practice (also see Ch.15). Meares believed that motivation to practice them was best achieved via suggestion in passing. He did this in his books and during informal conversation[136]. Comments like: "I knelt on the balcony at sunrise. It was very cold. The Stillness was deep" (said so you knew deep meant it felt so good you didn't really feel cold).[137] The suggestion was made and conversation naturally shifted onto the next topic. If rapport is sufficient, then identification and imitation do the rest.

Generic Examples

Examples can help communicate the kernel of an idea of what is involved. Generic examples provide a **starting point** to build on. Standing on someone's shoulders gives you a boost so you can go even higher. Such examples need to be customised to your own style, niche audience and setting, so they become both distinct and your own "same but different" approach to teaching Stillness Meditation.

---

[136] Personal observation *corroborated by others.*
[137] *Similar statements are also repeated throughout Meares' writings.*

1. Generic Benefits of Stillness Meditation

Reduced symptoms and sickness
- Reduced nervous symptoms. (SMSB Ch.4-8).
- Reduced bodily symptoms: *palpitation, upset gut (diarrhoea and rebound constipation), nervous urination, muscle tension & shakes, premature ejaculation, frigidity, insomnia.*
- Reduced nervous illness: *eg. phobias (snakes, insects, other) claustrophobia, agoraphobia, impotence etc.*
- Reduced psychosomatic illness: *dermatitis, asthma, headaches, high blood pressure, gut ulcers, premenstrual tension, ulcerative colitis.*
- Refer s2 regarding cancer and serious illness.
- Better coping with pain.
- Dignity in death if facing the reaper etc.

Benefits to work, study, family and relationships.
- Helps productivity, efficiency and creativity.
- Better concentration and improved decision-making.
- Allows intellect to be undistracted and undistorted.
- Earning capacity less held back.
- Also, see SMSB (Ch. 4-8, 10-12, 20-27).

Benefits for meaning, wellness and sports
- Enhanced sports performance plus better recovery.
- Enhances wordless prayer and the "spiritual" dimension.
- Science based anxiety reduction free of religious influence.
- Support factors (SMSB Ch. 9-18).
- Helps the individual psyche to evolve. (SMSB Ch. 4-8, 20-27):- includes things like altruism, compassion, empathy, mystic\ spiritual experience, intuition, meaning\ purpose and so on,
- Wellness to enable thriving, flourishing and enhanced resiliance.

Note: The benefits of anxiety reduction via Stillness Meditation are extensive. This list has gaps. Further information is provided in Ainslie Meares on Meditation and Still Mind Sound Body and, of course, in Dr Meares' writings from which those books were derived.

SMSB = Sound Mind Sound Body

© O Bruhn 2022

2. Generic Talk Topics

The teacher meets and talks to a group to help them get to know the teacher and learn about the benefits of reducing anxiety (refer generic example 1). Similar discussion may occur at registration meetings (see Ch 26.) and\or initial classes. A list of topics will help work out what areas to cover. The details and order depend upon niche, audience and purpose(s) of the talk.

- Life story about how the teacher came to learn Stillness Meditation. Things like:
  - Relevant life history.
  - Past occupational background.
  - Previous experience with therapies, if relevant.
  - Stillness meditation lineage.
  - Personal help experienced from Stillness Meditation.
- Explanation of Stillness Meditation (Ch. 2) eg
  - Symmetrical nonmoving position.
  - Pure effortless relaxation that spreads throughout body and mind.
  - Practised in slight discomfort.
  - Stillness of mind restores mental equilibrium and anxiety is reduced.
  - Cultivation of post meditative calm.
- Stillness Meditation vs other types (Ch. 3&5).
  - Stillness of mind rather than dullness of monotone[138] (mantra, breathing etc).
  - Reduction in anxiety due Stillness of mind.
  - Temporary regression to a simple mental state that rests and resets (or restores) the mind and body.
  - Slight discomfort (not comfort nor marked discomfort).
- Benefits relevant to your audience (refer previous page).
- Other topics relevant to teacher's story and/or client group.

---

[138] *Meares used both terms ie. dull and monotone.*

3. Generic Stillness Meditation Class
This is one example of "same but different" (refer Ch. 16).

Registration meeting
- Client meets with the teacher.
- After discussion, each client gives signed informed consent (see Ch. 25) to learn Stillness Meditation including touch (or is supported in waiving or deferring touch). Also, see "*Example Protocol Referencing Records*" in Ch. 26.
- Ideally, the client has read about Meares' approach. If not, then simple explanation is provided (together with motivation and rapport, as discussed earlier).
- This may be followed by a 1:1 Stillness Meditation session using verbal prompts and "the space between". If workable, in the same room used for Stillness Meditation class.

Group Session
Clients re-attend to participate as a group of 5-15:
- meditators arrive and seat themselves, close eyes and begin to relax. All arrived and seated.
- **5-10 mins.** The teacher meditates separately.
- **10 mins or so.** The teacher enters the Stillness Meditation room and uses verbal prompts and "the space between".
- **20 mins or so.** 1x round of shoulder touch followed by 1x round shoulders & head touch. "Round" means touch applied to each of the 10 meditators (ie. who had all consented to touch at registration).
- **15-20 mins.** Wake up and counter regression. Those known to counter regress quickly are seen and checked first.

Notes:
→ A smaller class size is easier to manage eg. 6 clients.
→ Clients provided presence and or touch as needed.
→ Rounds of touch depend upon class size.
→ Back up checks take longer with larger class size.
→ This example, including times, is purely indicative. No two sessions are ever identical. Nothing is rushed! Planning is essential if landlord imposed time limits exist.
→ An easy to read watch helps keep things calmly on schedule.

19. Therapeutic Touch

© O Bruhn 2022

Introduction

Therapeutic touch was discussed in S3. In this chapter, the biology of touch as it relates to calm and alarm is discussed. Next, an adjusted protocol for the non-medical use of therapeutic touch in modern times, is discussed. The reader will need to weigh up the risks and benefits of the use of therapeutic touch (see later).

Early Evolution of Touch

The first primordial cell had contact with its environment via its folding membranes. Then, in multicellular organisms there was contact between cells as well as the "without" of the external environment. In complex organisms, the sense of proprioception allows the organism to track limb position and movements. The sense of touch provides information about objects (or other organisms) that come into contact with the skin.

Touch is the oldest of the senses. It evolved into the other senses including taste, smell, vision and hearing.

Touch is direct. The other senses involve stimulus being transmitted via a medium (air) to the receiver. The pathway (gap) between stimulus and receiver remains although a signal is received. Touch detects a direct signal without any discernible gap.

Touch is the parent of smell, taste, vision and hearing. Not surprisingly, touch helps the other senses develop and if touch is neglected then the development of other senses is hindered.

Fight-Flight-Immobility

Nature selects out those who survive and have offspring. The unfit perish before mating or have fewer offspring. Instincts are built in support of evolution's inherent goals.

Potential danger alerts. This involves an instinctual pause, a motionless stop, which may be very brief in a calm person. This cessation of motion helps to decide which instinctual switch to flick. Statue like immobility also facilitates being ignored by an enemy, predator or prey. If one is immobile, distance, direction, and intention can be better estimated.

If danger abates (or opportunity to kill prey passes), then immobility settles into quiescent calm. Alternatively, immobility escalates to instinctual fight or flight.

Evolution selects animals designed to win. If that is not possible then to cut losses and live to breed another day. If instinct determines the fight is lost and flight is impossible, the loser may become immobile ie. faint or feign unconsciousness\death. A human victor might spare a defeated unconscious enemy. A predator might be fooled into letting go an untasty corpse. If able to do so, the loser flees, eventually hides and assumes instinctive silent immobility.

The win elates the victor. Another loser unable to flee has to make the best of defeat. Hiding in plain sight, may play a role in that too. The role of immobility itself, has also tended to be hidden in plain sight during discussions of fight and flight.

Reptiles and lower organisms are alerted into the fight-flight-immobility triad by proximity. But, mammals feed their young milk in proximity. Mammals had to evolve to over-ride proximity fight-flight[139]. This modified the fight-flight- immobility triad towards relative immobility while feeding and engaging in social grooming.

Young primates are fed, petted and kept warm by mother and provided warmth and social grooming by the group. The need for growth and development resulted in a longer relationship and more (non-sexual) touch between mother and young as well as within the group. Play can involve pushing, pulling, prodding, tickling of others as well as "touching" the environment. Some learning involves "not touching" sharp, hot or cold things. As well as learning taboos like avoiding touch that led to inbreeding or poisoning (eg. excreta).

Then further evolution occurred in our remote ancestors as additional verbal and nonverbal communication was built into this up close social touching. At some point, logic and critical thinking emerged. This also required a new type of rest from the intense mental activity. This occurred by allowing the mind to temporarily regress to the simple pre-verbal state of the remote ancestor.

The developmental sequence of babies involves touch, then auditory and the visual senses. In the development of language primitive touch helps build up auditory and visual signals and responses. Yet, in the development of close relationships, the older child or adult relates to others first through the visual and auditory sense and then touch. Even so, touch is subtly embedded in

---

139 Porges SW (2021), Polyvagal Theory: A biobehavioural journey to sociality, Comprehensive Psychoneuroendocrinology,V7.

language. *"That was rough"* *It felt smooth. It was hard. An abrasive person. They are soft."* We are urged *"to reach out"* and to *"handle them with care"* as we *"rubbed them the wrong way."* This all highlights the extent to which touch is a significant dimension in our lives *"connecting with others"*.

Having skimmed the literature on the evolution of touch we now turn to briefly skimming deficits and developmental defects (NB a bibliography is located at the end of this chapter).

Deficits & Developmental Faults

Human primitive cultures used touch to aid healing[140] and in the experience of the divine. Greek and Roman philosophers regarded touch as essential. Various rulers[141] deprived several children of their mothers and limited human contact to feeding, to reveal what language they first uttered. These diabolical experiments were gross failures usually put down to neglect. Yet, it might be said that a lack of both touch and lullabies is lethal or, at least, grossly debilitating.

Harlow's infamous experiments[142] describe how baby monkeys perished or were spectacularly psychologically damaged by cheap non-living substitutes for mother's touch.

The stories of wild children raised by animals go back to ancient times. Many seem genuine, some are hoaxes or attempts to disguise abuse. The children reared by animals often survive into adulthood although their language and behaviour is impaired.

Feral children is a term used to describe grossly abused children who endure years of maltreatment by parents or institutions. They usually survive to adulthood with impaired behaviour and language.

Broadly speaking, a failure to learn "social" touch results in:
- Social isolation.
- More alert and anxious with higher sympathetic basal tone.
- Tendency to be aggressive, run away and\or immobility.
- Impaired perception or processing of signals due to

---

140 Katz R (1982). Accepting "Boiling Energy".V10(4): 344-368; Marshall L (1969) The Medicine Dance of the Kung Bushmen. Africa: J Int African Inst 39(4):347-381; Thomas EM. The Harmless People. 1989; Johnston AE (1911). The Laying on of Hands. Irish Church Quarterly, 4(16):312–323; Smith HP (1913). The Laying-on of Hands. Amer J Theol, 17(1):47–62.
141 *Pharoah Psamtik I, Holy Roman Emperor Frederick II, James IV of Scotland and Mughal Emperor Akbar. Psamtik's victims are said to have uttered "bread" in Phrygian, which sounds like servants avoiding Pharoah's wrath.*
142 Harlow HF & Zimmermann RR (1958). The development of affective responsiveness in infant monkeys. Proc Amer Phil Soc 102:501-9; Harlow HF, Dodsworth RO & Harlow MK (1965).Total social isolation in monkeys. PNAS 54(1):90.

defective learning (as touch develops first and then helps the development of the other senses).
- Sensory overload arising from higher sympathetic tone due to high anxiety plus sensory modifications.

The range and severity of these deficits will vary depending upon the circumstances (ie. the neglect and lack of touch etc).

Our quick skim through evolution and literature makes it obvious that a lack of appropriate touch must harm. Next, we consider categories of touch.

Types of Touch

First, for clarity, we absolutely exclude those categories of touch that are NOT involved in Meares' protocol:
- Task-environment touch- contact points, proprioception.
- Playful touch such as prodding or tickling.
- Aggressive touching to abuse or threaten harm etc.
- Erotic touch to sexually arouse.

Touch in Meares' protocol is limited to the following:
- Conventional touch:
  - Greeting touch eg. shaking hands.
  - Orienting touch eg. steering by the shoulder or elbow.
  - Task-related touch eg. hands touch passing a paper, pen, medical exam, body worker exam and treatment etc. This also includes incidental touch during a task.
  - Assistance touch eg. help to stand or complete a task.
  - Attention-containment touch to gain attention if drowsy, to stop a person falling or walking into traffic.
- Therapeutic touch ie. calming touch to back, shoulders-upper chest, arms and head.
- Lawful touch to defend self or protect another.[143]

A Generic Protocol Aimed at Safer Touch

Principles
- Insurers, some psycho-analysts and drug prescribers refuse touch. This seems like unfamiliarity with, or denial of, the literature. *"Not to touch any clients at any time can be experienced as abusive as the original neglect to the... infant inside the adult client."*[144]

---

[143] *Included as a low probability event that might be realised one day.*
[144] Dr. Lubin-Alpert in Norwood, D. (2017 Jun 29). Touch in therapy: helpful or harmful? https://www.goodtherapy.org/blog/touch-in-therapy-helpful-or-harmful-

© O Bruhn 2022

- Touch is not inherently unethical. The evidence base (end of this chapter) urges ethical use of wanted and appropriate touch when it is likely to result in client benefits.
- **Conventional touch** means greeting, orienting task-related, assistance and attention-containment touch. Consent for conventional touch is provided by alignment with modern manners and culture. Conventional touch paves the way for therapeutic touch. The client's response to the former helps inform the process for the latter.
- Some psychotherapists substitute dogs for therapeutic touch. Wild children don't do as well as those with human parents. Pets would disrupt the meditation room and alarm clients with dog allergy (10%[145]) or cynophobia (10% [146]).
- Psychotherapists touch head, shoulders, back, arm and hands in verbal therapy.[147] Some ask for verbal consent before every touch! *May I shake you hand? May I steer you by the arm? May I take your arm to stop you falling? May I shift the position of my hand on your shoulder?* When does one touch stop and the next begin? *My hand is on your shoulder, is that still OK?* The client may feel the above approach as cold and insensitive. This inhibits rapport that allows facilitation of calm. Asking for consent prior to each therapeutic touch would alert meditators away from calm, breach privacy and result in substandard care. Prior informed consent needs to be obtained at registration.
- The teacher stands in a senior position in a professional relationship with the client. This results in rapport and acts to prevent inappropriate relationships. A work "uniform" reinforces an expectation of a formal professional relationship. It includes dressing in a clean, professional, non-revealing manner with minimal scent and jewellery.
- Skin infection is not mentioned in the touch literature, nor by those who deny touch nor in mental health worker codes. Non-medical therapeutic touch is to back, shoulders, upper chest, arms and head of clothed meditators. Keep hands clean as per activities of daily living.[148] Don't touch visibly

---

one-therapists-perspective-0629175. accessed 2022.
145 https://www.healthdirect.gov.au/cat-and-dog-allergy. Accessed end 2022.
146 *10% population v. approx based on unreferenced data on reputable websites.*
147 Zur O & Nordmarken N (undated) To Touch Or Not To Touch. https://www.zurinstitute.com/resources/touch-in-therapy/ accessed end 2022.
148 NHMRC (2022). Aust. Guidelines for Prevention and Control of Infection in Health Care. *Included for those dealing with unusual client groups.*

- abnormal skin unless infection has been excluded [See Ch. 25 for infected teacher obligations].
- Some doctors use a nurse observer for the medical exam. Unlike patients, meditators are fully clothed and therapeutic touch is restricted to back, shoulders-upper chest, arms and head. It is unviable for a second meditation teacher[149] to observe a 1 hr class with up to 15 clients. The use of an observer in a class would need unanimous consent agreed by all meditators. A fixed security camera, might act as an observer. A portable camera would provoke complaints ie. privacy,"creepy" etc. The group of meditators themselves act as observers to an extent.
- Protocols, training and seeking help from colleagues can help reduce the probability of error but won't eliminate it. Touch involves feeling. Mistakes can occur. The teacher, client or both may inadvertently contribute to mistakes. Third parties may contribute to mistakes or errors, too.

Touch is Discussed at Registration
- The client is informed about Stillness Meditation eg. touch to back, shoulders-upper chest, arms and head whilst seated and fully clothed. Large hands placed on small shoulders may result in finger tips draped beyond the inferior clavicular border onto the upper chest.
- A confidential client history is sought to identify any reasons to defer touch (eg. past sexual or physical abuse, gender related issues, culture or religious belief[150], other). If the client seems reticent, they are encouraged to defer touch.
- Signed consent is obtained or deferred. The client is empowered to defer or request touch later. Avoiding confusion means there can't be many changes.
- Stillness Meditation may be facilitated without touch at registration and this might be done for an initial class session if all clients are "beginners".

Identifying Touch Consent In Class (Options)
- **A mixed group.** The teacher provides touch only to clients who have given informed consent.

---

149 *Untrained observers can't be used eg.* Health Complaints Commissioner Vic. vs Weinstein\CDC Clinics Pty Ltd (several). *Allegations existed, at least in part, as an unqualified manager entering the consultation room.*

150 *Several religions\cultures prohibit touching opposite sex, head, or by left hand and some completely prohibit touch*

© O Bruhn 2022

- **Designated areas for those to sensitive to allow touch.** Client's who have not consented to touch sit in a signposted designated area\chairs. An error might occur if a client sits in the wrong seat. Steering clients to a specific seat could avoid that but requires the teacher to recall each client's consent status.
- **Non-touch classes.** All new clients attend initial classes without touch (Number specified by teacher). Next, those consenting to touch progress to sessions with touch. Those having waived touch continue on without touch. This approach presupposes it is viable to run several classes. It may result in client's feeling they are missing out or requests to swap classes with touch status unchanged (eg. client convenience).
- Other approaches are possible (eg. hovering hands).

Delivery of Therapeutic Touch

- The teacher pauses at the client's chair so that a dim awareness dawns on the client. The ideal timing results in the client expecting touch before it arrives.
- Touch is delivered, to the best of the teacher's ability to communicate calm and to avoid alerting. This involves feelings rather than black and white logic. If the teacher feels an unintended client response, they modify delivery of that touch ie via adjusting timing and delivery to reduce closeness ie. increase "the space between" so touch calms rather than alerts.
- Refer Ch 12 & 13.

Note 1. Modern manners and culture assist task related touch yet, consent requirements exist in various occupational codes of conduct. Hence, this generic protocol may need to be modified for individual circumstances.

Note 2. The reader needs to carefully consider their own situation and weigh up the risks and benefits of touch. Where touch is used, the adopted process should be documented to show workability and the impracticality of alternatives. This may not prevent concerns or complaints being raised but, it does enable documentation to be made available for 3rd party verification, if required.

Brief Bibliography on Touch

1. Ardiel EL, Rankin CH. The importance of touch in development. Paediatr Child Health. 2010 Mar;15(3):153-6.
2. Barnett L (2005) Keep in touch: The importance of touch in infant development. Infant Observation. August 2005, 1-17
3. Cascio CJ, Moore S, McGlone F (2019) Social touch and human development. Developmental Cognitive Neuroscience. 35: 5-11.
4. Carlson M, Earls F (1997). Psychological and neuroendocrine sequelae of early social deprivation in institutionalized children in Romania. Ann NY Acad Sci. Jan 15;807:419-28.
5. Deangelis T & Mwakalyelye N (1995). The power of touch helps vulnerable babies thrive. APA Monitor, Oct 25.
6. Field T. (2001). Touch. Cambridge MA. (incl Fields 1999a&b).
7. Field, T. (2010). Touch for socioemotional and physical well-being: A review. Developmental Review, 30(4), 367-383.
8. Newton M (2004) Savage Girls and Wild Boys.
9. Porges SW (https://www.everydayhealth.com/wellness/united-states-of-stress/advisory-board/stephen-w-porges-phd-q-a/)
10. Porges SW. (1995) Orienting in a defensive world. Psychophysiology. 32(4):301-18.
11. Porges, SW (2021). Cardiac vagal tone: a neurophysiological mechanism that evolved in mammals to dampen threat reactions and promote sociality. World Psychiatry, 20(2): 296.
12. Porges SW (2022) Polyvagal Theory: A Science of Safety. Frontiers in Integrative Neuroscience 16.
13. Roelofs K (2017). Freeze for action: neurobiological mechanisms in animal and human freezing. Phil Trans R Soc B 372: 20160206.
14. Therapeutic Touch Int. Assoc. (2018). Bibliography on therapeutic touch https://therapeutictouch.org/about-us/research/. *Practiced by either direct contact or at a short distance. Included for general information.*
15. Rovers M, Maletter J, Guirguis-Younger M (2017) Touch in the Helping Professions. University of Ottawa Press.
16. Zur O (2007). Touch in Therapy and the Standard of Care in Psychotherapy and Counseling. USABPJ. 6. 61-93.
17. Zur O & Nordmarken N To Touch Or Not To Touch. https://www.zurinstitute.com/resources/touch-in-therapy/ accessed 2022.
18. Zur O. Ethical and Legal Aspects of Touch in Psychotherapy https://www.zurinstitute.com/resources/touch-in-therapy/ accessed 2022.

© O Bruhn 2022

20. Venue Design & Selection

Introduction

Translating Meares' approach into the modern teaching situation depends upon niche audience, setting and venue (eg.dedicated or shared). Different situations need different arrangements. Thought is needed on how a natural and calming situation can be created within the applicable constraints. Flexibility is needed as some things may be changed and others not.

Some Stillness Meditation teachers already have a venue and client niche. They may not be able to modify the building much but, may be able to change how it is utilised.

Other Stillness Meditation teachers have neither venue nor client group. They can choose, within budget, what they lease, rent or purchase. For long term lease, minor renovation may be an option. (NB Leases usually require that modifications are approved by the landlord and "made good" at tenant's cost at the end of the lease.)

At Home

A large house <u>may</u> be able to be adapted to Stillness Meditation teaching in line with building and local council requirements (ie. activity permitted in zone, signage & facilities). Separate access for client's is a good idea, if council, house design and budget permit.

An early conversation with neighbours will help avoid designing in problems. This is cheaper than revising application's or making structural changes later. Neighbours may have no concerns and appreciate the transparency. Any specifics can be identified, discussed and considered. The local council (see later) can advise on requirements etc. that may apply to your home and proposed usage.

Aside from uncooperative neighbours there are further considerations. If one had shockingly bad luck one might acquire a client who became a pest. A preventive attitude might lead one to conclude that home might not be the best option. In a previous role, I learnt that many people's residential address can be tracked down. Many people (not limited to Stillness Mediation teachers) prefer to separate workplace from home and also use a PO Box address. This neatly leads into consideration of alternatives.

Lease, Hire or Rental

Other options are to hire, rent or lease a suitable venue. Potential venues include scout-guide halls, churches, community centres, school halls, recreation/ sporting clubs, commercial or other venues.

Walk around the perimeter of the planned venue. Also, do a walk through **inspection** of the venue **at the time(s) you plan to rent** to avoid problems (also see Ch. 26). Examples include:
- Isolated unlit areas with "undesirables" loitering versus cars parked in a well lit open area next to lockable entrance.
- Activities that might interrupt eg. loud disruptive noises next door, persons opening or knocking on doors or walls.
- Conditions eg. slips, trips, falls, traffic and unsafe chairs.

Would be landlords want to avoid problems too. Some worry that "alternative therapies" may involve property damaging rituals or complaints from neighbours. You can reassure them that Stillness Meditation involves a small silent group sitting on chairs enjoying intense peace and quiet. Be prepared to provide qualifications, insurance held (Ch. 26) etc.

Religious Landlords. Some churches prohibit religious meditative practices. It will be necessary to explain that Stillness Meditation is non-religious and can be practised independently of or alongside Christian (or some other) religions. In theory, some atheist or sceptic landlords might need convincing of an absence of link between Stillness Meditation and religion or doctrine.

Building Code, Planning & Bylaws

You should check that any venue you propose to purchase, lease or rent complies with Building Code, Planning and Local By Laws. The local council, fee-for-service building surveyor or an architect can advise on occupancy (numbers of people, permitted use), toilet facilities (inside or close by) and other requirements, if present. You may also be able to ask the landlord to see the occupancy permit (or certificate of final inspection).

You can identify the relevant council via the address and postcode of the proposed venue. If the premises is on a boundary road then the councils can tell you which one of them is responsible. In 2023, the links below provided council boundary information:

NSW www.olg.nsw.gov.au/ or www.screen.nsw.gov.au/page/maps
NT nt.gov.au/community/local-councils-remote-communities-and-homelands/maps-of-shires,-councils-and-local-authorities
QLD results.ecq.qld.gov.au/local_area_maps/
SA www.lga.sa.gov.au/sa-councils/councils-listing
TAS www.lgat.tas.gov.au/data/assets/pdf_file/0027/322983/ Local_Govt_Area_A4_map.pdf
VIC www.vec.vic.gov.au/ElectoralBoundaries/LocalCouncilMaps.html
    or knowyourcouncil.vic.gov.au

WA mycouncil.wa.gov.au/

Venue Elements

Teaching Stillness Meditation in modern times may involve arrangements that vary from Meares' medical clinic. Desirable functional requirements are:
- A reception and or greeting area.
- An area for the preliminary meeting (registration).
- A separate area for solo teacher meditation before class starts.
- A Stillness Meditation Room with suitable chairs.
- A debrief area.
- Toilet and hand washing facilities (in building or close by).
- Record management (digital or hard copy).

The simplest combination of core elements is:
- A room used for registration and Stillness Meditation (that doubles as an office).
- An adjacent area used for reception, greeting, debriefing and solo teacher meditation.

A registration meeting in the same premises as classes are held allows the client to rehearse the journey to and through the venue, and into the Stillness Meditation room. This will help client confidence on return to their first group class. If renting a venue for only the duration of Stillness Meditation class, a digital registration meeting might be needed (Ch. 21).

Other factors, like client safety and security (see earlier), car parking, proximity to public transport and located close to area(s) where interested clients will be drawn from are also desirable.

Greeting, Reception & Debrief Areas

In larger venues, **reception may be staffed by venue personnel**. The teacher will need to consider what they can allocate to venue staff and what they need to do themselves. This may also be set out in rental agreements. The agreement may allow some room to move.

The teacher greets clients as they arrive and debriefs them, after Stillness Meditation, at convenient point(s) (eg. waiting room, foyer or even adjacent to the Stillness Meditation room). Greeting and debrief might be at the same or separate points. More than one arrangement might be viable in the same multi room venue. In some instances, the layout allows:
- Clients enter through the main entrance.
- Greeted near or at the entrance to the Stillness Meditation

room after walking down a foyer or corridor, and
- Post Stillness Meditation departing via another door inside the meditation room. Debrief then occurs at that door or just outside it with the remaining meditators inside.

In other instances, there is **no venue staffed reception**. The teacher then undertakes all functions ie. reception, greeting and debrief. These might be undertaken at the same or separate points. More than one arrangement may be viable in the same venue.

So far as is workable, these points should have visual and acoustic separation that results in privacy. Acoustic privacy helps to ensure the client is not reticent to disclose any concerns. Visual privacy may be tested by use of line of sight. Acoustic privacy is best tested by the help of assistants with good hearing. Distance and barriers (eg. closing doors) etc. may also be involved.

A single roomed building or hall. The single room is used for Stillness Meditation. Other functions:
- Reception\greeting near the entrance. The Stillness Meditation area is at the far end. The distance being such that conversations can't be overheard. A sound test with assistants will verify. If that doesn't work then reception may need to be just outside the entrance.
- Debrief just outside the entrance as the remaining meditators are inside the hall

Teacher solo meditation just before class starts. This might be in an adjacent room, a quiet corridor or even a corner of the Stillness Meditation room at a pinch.

The Stillness Meditation Room

Meares shifted rooms from time to time. So, he had more than one Stillness Meditation room but, they shared common properties.

Conspicuous Identification

Ideally, the layout will be such that the access and location of the Stillness Meditation room will be obvious to the client. In dedicated facilities, the room can be sign posted. In temporary facilities, where there is mixed usage a removable sign may be used. At some point, Meares sign posted his Stillness Meditation room *"The Quiet Place"*. A name with inherent subliminal cues. Peace and quiet.

Chair & Layout

Wing backed chairs. The chairs in Meares' *Quiet Place* were placed in rows, facing in one direction. Meares selected large leather Victorian wing backed chairs as they created a partial visual barrier between patients. The large flat back "shielded" the back of the patient sitting in it so, they can't be seen from behind. On side view, sitting in such a chair one can't see faces of adjacent people. A wisp of hair, a hand, or sleeve may be just visible. The seated patient had privacy. They were not alone and were part of a group.

Minimalist chairs. Today, fashion has moved on and people are used to a more minimal chair at gatherings. If workable, some variation in chair size and height is useful. One or two solid chairs with a high safe working load are useful for overweight clients. Chair stability is another factor.

The layout and access to the Stillness Meditation room needs to consider the privacy of the client including the direction they will be facing when seated. Ideally, the entry point should be towards the side or rear so that clients can arrive unobtrusively. This also meets a universal mental stereotype for seated gatherings eg. churches, theatres etc. It allows individual clients to be debriefed afterwards from the rear row forwards which also fosters a sense of privacy. Although, the order of client debrief may vary as those who wake up quickly are seen first.

Seat selection. Meares' seated each patient. Someimes, there was a short queue of people waiting their turn at the front door. Another approach is to greet people at the entrance and allow them to seat themselves. The layout of the premises being used, particularly in multi roomed venues may make this approach desirable (also see earlier).

Space between chairs. The teacher should check the arrangement of chairs prior to each class. Adequate space between chairs is needed to avoid the teacher tripping over chairs or personal items brought into the room by clients, like handbags etc. Clients should be instructed to place personal items underneath chairs. If there is insufficient space then these items will need to be secured at another location to avoid a slip, trip situation. Also, check adequate clearance (0.8 m) between chair backs and walls to allow delivery of touch.

Allow sufficient access between the front of the chair seat in one row and the back of the chairs in the next ie. to allow for the lower limbs of seated clients so the teacher is be able to safely pass by. 1.25 m approx. may suffice. The size of the room may result in some constraints which won't apply in a hall. In a hall, the chairs should **not be spread too far apart**, to avoid loss of a sense of being a group within the protective influence of the teacher.

Avoiding a sprain, strain or injury from slip or trips etc. is obvious when considering layout and tidiness. A slip or trip (or recovery) is alerting. The smooth relaxed motion of the teacher through uncluttered layout and tidiness signals relaxation to clients.

Prior to the pandemic, a water jug, cups and tissues were accessible in the Stillness Meditation room. Plastic jug and glasses will help avoid any potential for broken glass, such as might occur during access by a tense or drowsy participant. A bin fitted with a bag to contain used tissues etc. will help avoid direct handling.

Aesthetic items might be added to the Stillness Meditation room, especially if on long term lease or owned by the teacher. Any additions are suggested to be streamlined and minimal.

Airborne Infectious Disease

Chapter 26 discusses OHS and related matters to be considered during the design and selection of a venue (eg.evacuation etc). It seems that airborne infectious disease like COVID-19, flu and others are with us to stay. Some tips:

- Keep up to date with the applicable local requirements. Local rules may vary and change over time.
- Some landlords specify airborne infection related rules on rental or lease documents.
- Adequate ventilation ie. room air changes per hour. Air circulation in ordinary rooms is never homogeneous. Being upwind near known fresh air inlets is of benefit.
- Correctly fitted P2\N95 masks substantially reduce the number of airborne microbes inhaled. Removing them for short periods significantly reduces the protection factor.
- Coughing throws fine aerosols a substantial distance (10 metres or so) before natural air movement takes over.
- Clean frequently touched surfaces with a sanitiser. Use a personal hand sanitiser before class (and afterwards).
- Precautions for COVID-19 susceptible clients depend on local laws etc. and may include negative RAT tests and so on.
- For requirements if teacher becomes infected refer Ch. 25.

If masks are to be worn inside, an outdoor greeting will let the teacher see client's faces and assess demeanour. Clients close their eyes at the start of Stillness Meditation. So, a mask donned by the teacher would not be seen. On arrival, clients would need to be informed, and some may need to be reminded, that you intend to don a mask to avoid any who sneaked a peak tensing up in surprise.

21. A Digital Venue

© O Bruhn 2022

The Birth of Digital Meetings

The internet was an embryo at the time Meares' passed and "Apps" were unknown. Skype started in 2005. At the start of the COVID-19 pandemic, "telehealth" took off. Health practitioners welcomed remote consultations that stopped exposure to COVID-19. Digital meetings became widespread. However, telehealth is new and with no widely agreed tested legal standards but, many continue with digital meetings. It is convenient. It avoids costs of commuting\travel, parking and renting rooms. It allows teacher and client to be anywhere and meet at any time. Those in remote or unusual locations can attend (eg. farmers, ships, prisons etc). The OHS and SHC Agencies(see later, Ch. 23), use this technology themselves. There is not yet much guidance on precautions required for legal compliance and safe use. This will change and may do so quickly without warning.

The Physical Stillness Meditation Room

The situation in the physical Stillness Meditation room is clear enough. Both teacher and clients are physically present together in the same room. The "space between" and wanted touch may be utilised. The teacher is able to act quickly in an emergency (eg. heart attack etc), render assistance and summon further help (calling 000 and so on) (see Ch. 26).

The Digital Stillness Meditation Room

The situation is different in a digital meeting. There are unknowns and potential concerns (not limited to):
- Ability to verify the clients' identity, age and location. Emphasis on a thorough registration meeting.
- Digital attendance when client wouldn't physically attend:
  - Drug\alcohol usage, harder to detect (eg. won't see drunk walk\sway or smell breath).
  - Observable injury or bruises?
  - Unwell.
  - Under duress.
- Limitations of digital group Stillness Meditation sessions:

- Nonverbal communication is nearly eliminated.
- The calm community of the group may not be evoked to the extent as when all present in a physical room.
• Responding to difficulties during session (eg. heart attack):
  - Client location known and accurate?
  - Emergency contacts? Australian 000 system is state based If you ring 000 in Victoria they send help to Vict. 000 won't work outside Australia. emergency numbers may be local, state or national - it differs from country to country.
• Counter regression. Camera views are of face, not usually of motion and gait. More reliance on verbal discussion.
• Disrupted or failed communication during Stillness Meditation, at time of emergency or before counter regression. A second line of communication is needed in case the primary means can't be restored. Client is advised to set a back up independent timer alarm for end of session.
• Digital security measures that protect teacher and client data from third party access or disclosure.
• Legal requirements on teacher may differ in client jurisdictions. Two jurisdictions apply.
• New technology and differing situations may reveal further risks that can't be discussed as they are presently unknown. Yet, all potential hazards need to be identified, risks assessed and actions put into place to ensure risks are adequately controlled.

Some risks can be reduced by restricting digital teaching to client's well known to the teacher who already have an established meditation practice. Yet, risk remains not limited to actual client location, emergency contacts and jurisdictional requirements. Other unidentified risks may be present. Some of them will seem obvious in hindsight! Decades of OHS experience make it clear that requirements may change rapidly as further guidance is provided by regulatory agencies or the courts via "case law" (set by prosecution).

CDs, Apps & So On

Some teachers of Stillness Meditation have made CDs to help clients practice at home. However, the general advice is to abandon all such aids as soon as possible. One wants to be able to experience Stillness whenever and wherever one decides to practice. Aids impose unwanted limits and can become a crutch. Besides, once the mind is still you won't hear the CD, anyway.

© O Bruhn 2022

22. Interfacing With Other Methods

Introduction

Effortless relaxation involves less. Passing from the waking state to Stillness of mind involves a passive lessening. Meares' method is already simple, direct and efficient. The inclusion of unrelated elements adds complexity, dilution and inefficiency.

Today, doctors, nurses, therapists, body workers, tai chi teachers, school teachers, psychologists, HR professionals, ministers, counsellors, artists and others[151] teach Stillness Meditation. My own centre point is Meares' Stillness Meditation, yet I also utilise other methods. In all cases, there is a fine dividing line between Stillness Meditation and other methods.

The examples below of physical activity and Stillness Meditation help to illustrate how to meet goals and avoid crossing that fine line.

Physical Activity & Stillness Meditation

Keep Risk Low, Safety First

Too little physical activity is a risk, as is too much. The aim is to straighten and strengthen rather than weaken and injure! Before beginning any exercise program **get health practitioner clearance**. If your doctor says it's OK, then, use perfect form and **stop any exercise, if pain occurs**.

Meares' Morning Recharge

Our starting point is Dr Ainslie Meares' morning recharge mentioned in Ch. 9. It is briefly summarised below:
1. Stillness Meditation for 10 mins or so.
2. A leisurely walk in the park.

Meares' "meditate and walk" approach emphasises the onflow of calm and ease. Clearly, this combination of time spent in Stillness followed by cultivation of onflow is very important in starting the day if teaching, or not. This approach may be followed 7 days a week.

The Author's 2020-2022 Recharge

Today, healthful physical activity involves alignment, straightening and strengthening the body, as well as gait based activity. Alignment at the start of the day, helps take better posture

---
[151] *Apologies to any professions I forgot to mention!*

into daily life. Time may be limited and a short physical "recharge" is can be in parallel with the mental recharge.

Pandemic lockdown stopped walking and the author's[152] recharge is described below. Asterisked* exercises are described elsewhere[153].

1. **Stillness Meditation** in *static back,* 10 mins or so.
2. * *Standing arm circle*   50/50 each way.
3. *Elbow curls*   25 reps.
4. *Overhead extension*(see footnote[154])   30 sec
5. **Marching**   60-100 reps
(knees to 90 degrees, arms move in sagittal plane).

Exercises 2-4 require about 3 minutes. Marching can be set at the same duration as the walk. These days a walk or *function run,* an aligned relaxed jog, may be done instead as there is no lockdown.

A physical and mental workout – 5MBX+

In the early 1970s, Meares wrote 5MX[155] (5 Mental Exercises). At that time, the 5 body exercise (5BX) Canadian Air Force plan[156] had become very popular. Meares suggested that 5BX could be practiced with Stillness Meditation (5MX), but left how it might be done up to the reader. By way of tribute to Dr Meares' work and to provide a further example, 5MX is interfaced with 5BX below.

Adding postural alignment at the start of 5BX prepares the body for work. After the work unwanted postural compensations are removed and alignment is restored which prepares the body to return to daily living. This makes it 5MBX plus (aka "5MBX+"). The *asterisked** exercises are described elsewhere[157].

Two versions of 5MBX+ for use near the start of the day are outlined below:

If wide awake:
1. **Stillness Meditation** for 10 mins or so in *static back* (which also provides simple pre-workout alignment).
2. 5BX Level 1: toe touch, sit up, back raise, push up & run. (or run in place, refer "100-up-exercise" in footnote[158])
3. *Air Bench (30sec to 1 min).*

If slow to wake up:

---

152 *Derived from a sequence created by Brian Bradley, Egoscue specialist.*
153 Still Mind Sound Body
154 From Crooked Body to Joints in Line. *Available from internet retailers.*
155 Meares A. Life Without Stress. Appendix 5MX. 1987. pp121-128.
156 5BX Plan for Physical Fitness Royal Canadian Air Force. 1961. https://csclub.uwaterloo.ca/~rfburger/5bx-plan.pdf. Accessed end 2022.
157 Still Mind Sound Body
158 https://starkcenter.org/exhibits/type/digital-resources/the-100-up-exercise/ Acessed end 2022.

© O Bruhn 2022

1. *Cat Dog 10 rep then * Counter stretch 1 min.
2. 5BX sequence.
3. **Stillness Meditation** for 10 mins or so in *static back*.

Those with a history of back pain or a doctor who says "no" to 5BX might ask if a sequence from Ch. 14 in Still Mind Sound Body might be OK (also review "Keep Risks Low, Safety First").

Meares[159] wrote Stillness Meditation may be before, after or unrelated to exercise. An uncommon approach might involve a Stillness Meditation sandwich eg. before and after another activity.

Meares' "meditate and walk" approach emphasises the cultivation of the onflow of calm and ease. Alternatively, an approach like the author's pandemic recharge might be used. Essentially, "meditate, align & walk".

In the morning, if one is sleepy then physical activity can help wake up first and that will help Stillness Meditation. If you feel fatigued from mental activity, later in the day, then one may relax into calm before exercising. If the workout is arduous causing mental or physical fatigue then one can meditate afterwards.

Gaps between taxing physical "workouts" require sufficient time for adaptation. Fitness improvement depend upon recovery. "Workouts" (eg. 5MBX+ or similar) might be done 3-5 days/week with a morning "mediate and walk" 7 days/week, which can be done twice a day on the days taxing workouts aren't done, if desired.

Static Back. Static back allows gravity to settle and align the neck, shoulders, spine and hips. In Meares' lifetime, static back was unknown. It is a *symmetrical, slightly uncomfortable position*[160] that resembles sitting on a chair but laying down. Stillness Meditation in static back can be undertaken just as in any of the meditation positions in Meares' posture progression. It offers advantages to those meditators in pain (eg.hip or back pain) or sick (eg.worn down by cancer). For those interested in a morning "recharge" it is a more efficient use of time ie allows Stillness Meditation whilst passive alignment occurs in the background. If Meares had known of static back, in my opinion, he would have included it as an option in his posture progression.

Interface by Sequencing & Separation

Meares' atavistic regression theory of mental homeostasis forms the basis of Stillness Meditation teaching (see Ch. 3). His book, The Management of the Anxious Patient, discusses the application of the atavistic regression theory to psycho-social therapies. Do note that

---

159 Meares A (1989) A Better Life. pp68-69
160 *Meares' criteria for meditation postures. Refer* Ainslie Meares on Meditation.

some other methods are incompatible with Stillness Meditation. For example, other types of meditation are out as they involve subtle effort, active mental states, in some cases comfort and so on.

Some other activities with distinct goals are compatible sequenced with Stillness Meditation eg. the physical activity examples discussed above.

S3 emphasised rapport formed and built from the time of first greeting with explanation kept separate from Stillness Meditation. Chapter 18 discussed how explanation and motivation fit in. Explanation, motivation and rapport are used freely during many other activities. But, towards the fine dividing line (or interface) rapport predominates and is then exclusively utilised as Stillness Meditation commences. Understanding these principles also helps correctly position the fine dividing line between Stillness Meditation and other activities.

Teaching Stillness Meditation "same but different" was discussed earlier (Ch. 16). Stillness Meditation <u>appropriately</u> interfaced with another method might be thought of as "same but different". However, we can go further and say that interfacing also requires "sequence & separate".

A clear understanding of both methods ensures sequencing that supports the aims. This in turn helps identify the dividing line that results in an interface that separates Stillness Meditation from another method. The result being a relatively seamless process in which rapport predominates and becomes the exclusive communication before the fine dividing line after which Stillness Meditation commences. If the other activity is to be undertaken after Stillness Meditation then consideration needs to be given to allowing meditators sufficient time to undergo counter regression. For example, to comprehend explanation planned to be provided.

© O Bruhn 2022

S5. Providing a Health Service

Author's note: This section was completed in Victoria, in 2022. Checks by the reader are needed as applicable laws and standards vary by location, change over time, and professional bodies, insurers and regulators each hold their own interpretation as to what is applicable and constitutes compliance. The best check is an informed legal opinion. If you operate outside of Australia live or in the digital environment checks with local authorities are critical.

© O Bruhn 2022

23. Meditation Teaching is a Health Service

Introduction

Ainslie Meares, MD spent decades working as a medical specialist. He reflexively addressed ethical and administrative aspects. These things were at his fingertips. Meares' main concern was spreading Stillness Meditation- his gift to humanity. Some people he taught went on to teach Stillness Meditation themselves. Some of the new teachers had a professional background that acquainted them with ethical and administrative matters. Others had to learn these things for themselves.

The chapters in this section (S5) provide some assistance to those less experienced in such matters. First and foremost, this book is about teaching Stillness Meditation rather than a "business book". So, it was critical to avoid skewing the balance. To avoid that, S5 outlines some (but not all) general principles and instead points to further sources of information.

This chapter outlines some categories of health service providers. It sketches the Australian National and State adopted legislative framework that applies to those who teach meditation.

AHPRA Registered Health Practitioners

"AHPRA registered practitioners" are regulated by the Aust. Health Practitioner Registration Agency (www.ahpra.gov.au)[161]. AHPRA documentation sets the scope for work covered by registration. An AHPRA registered practitioner who operates outside their scope set by AHPRA must also comply with separate provisions as they are deemed "non AHPRA" providers. **This includes AHPRA registered practitioner who teach meditation.**

---

161 *At end 2022, registered professions include: Aboriginal & Torres Strait islander health practice, Chinese medicine, chiropractic, dentistry, medicine, medical radiation, nursing & midwifery, occupational therapy, optometry, osteopathy, paramedicine, pharmacy, physiotherapy, podiatry, and psychology practitioners.*

"Non AHPRA" Providers

In 2015, all Australian States endorsed a National Code of Conduct (National Code) that applies to "non AHPRA" providers.[162] Meditation Teachers were amongst many groups specifically mentioned as being covered[163]. Ch. 25 (see Mandatory Referral) briefly outlines the many other occupational roles also covered. The general approach of the National Code includes:

- #Safe, culturally sensitive and ethical services.
- #Informed consent.
- Appropriate conduct in relation to treatment advice.
- Appropriately response to adverse events.
- #Keeping appropriate records and comply with privacy laws.
- #Appropriate insurance.
- #Making available access to Code and how to complain.
- Standard precautions for infection control.
- #Modifying (or ceasing) providing if health, infection, or prescribed drugs place clients at risk.
- No false claims or misinformation about "quals" or services.
- No claims to cure certain serious illnesses.
- Not providing services under influence of alcohol or drugs.
- Not to financially exploit clients.
- #Not to engage in sexual misconduct.
- #Mandatory referral requirements.
  # Further guidance was to be made available for hash (#) marked points but none as at end 2022[164].

The State Health Complaint Agencies (SHC Agencies; see below) have each made laws (SHC Law) to give effect to the National Code:

- ACT: Human Rights Commission.
  www.hrc.act.gov.au/health

---

[162] National Code of Conduct for health care workers. COAG Health Council 2015.
[163] Final Report. National Code of Conduct for health care workers. COAG Health Council 2015. pg 52.
[164] Final Report. National Code of Conduct for health care workers. COAG Health Council 2015. pg 71. ...*many respondents to the consultation highlighted the need for support materials to be made available... The following clauses... were highlighted... as requiring clarification by... explanatory materials...* [Refer to cross hatched (#) points listed in list in body of book text]. *It is proposed that nationally consistent materials be produced by and the content mutually agreed by all...The materials would explain...the obligations... under the National Code. Explanatory notes would provide context for each of the clauses.*

- NT: Health and Community Services Complaints Commission. www.hcscc.nt.gov.au
- NSW: Health Care Complaints Commission. www.hccc.nsw.gov.au
- Qld: Office of the Health Ombudsman. www.oho.qld.gov.au
- SA: Health and Community Services Complaints Commission. www.hcscc.sa.gov.au
- Tas. Health Complaints Commission www.healthcomplaints.tas.gov.au
- WA. Health and Disability Services Complaints Office www.hadsco.wa.gov.au
- Vic. Health Complaints Commissioner www.hcc.vic.gov.au

The resulting SHC Laws vary somewhat from the National Code[165]. A 2022 Code (30 pages) that includes much additional guidance covers most AHPRA practitioners[166]. The National Code is 4 pages long. A lack of explanatory material makes it harder to identify detailed standards. Checks may be needed for details. These will need to be repeated if concerns were raised.

Occupation And Obligation

School Teachers

School teachers are registered to teach by State Institutes of Teaching (called boards or colleges in some States). If school teachers also teach meditation they do so as health service providers. School teachers were not intended to be exempt from SHC Law[167].

Religious Meditation Teaching

Human rights and equal opportunity laws support religious freedom to the boundary that it must not impinge upon any of the human rights of others. The situation for religious meditation teachers is similar to that of school teachers. There is no exemption for religious meditation teaching from SHC Law[168].

---

165 *For example, Victoria has complaint handling standards, duty of candour & health service principles, in addition, to its version of the National Code (Sched. 2).*
166 AHPRA. Revised Shared code of conduct.June 2022.
167 Final Report. National Code of Conduct for health care workers. COAG Health Council 2015. *Comments indicate that health education services were intended to be included and SHC Law in several States explicitly mentions them.*
168 Final Report. National Code of Conduct for health care workers. COAG Health Council 2015. *This report states to the effect that COAG intended that the Code apply to spiritual and esoteric healing practices (not limited to religious meditation teaching pg 26), yoga pg52 and also refer elsewhere in report.*

AHPRA Registered Practitioners

AHPRA registered practitioners teaching meditation must comply with SHC Law as meditation teaching is (nearly always) outside the scope of their AHPRA registration.

Miscellaneous

Meditation Teachers without professional affiliation need to comply with SHC Law.

Meditation teachers affiliated with Meditation Australia must comply with both Meditation Australia Codes and SHC Law.

Those with professional affiliations, like school teachers, religious meditation teachers and AHPRA registered practitioners, must follow the rules of the professional bodies in which they retain membership as well as SHC Law. Omission of a requirement in one set means complying with the other. If there were a gap or conflict between professional body rules and SHC Law then that would need to be reconciled. Some people who are members of several such associations will need to work out their, possibly unique, set of obligations.

In any of the above cases, if doubt exists, seek further advice.

Those teaching in a digital meditation room may be teaching in dual (or several) jurisdictions (ie. teaching and client's locations). In Australia, teaching across State boundaries will involve 2 or more sets of SHC Law plus professional association obligations. Overseas will involve the applicable jurisdictions rules plus professional association obligations.

SHC Law is unusual in that it picks up on privacy, health records, anti-discrimination, finance, insurance, qualifications and some other matters. Other laws also apply and some but not all of them are mentioned in subsequent chapters.

Definitions

AHPRA. Aust. Health Practitioner Registration Agency.
National Code of Conduct for Health Care Workers.
SHC Agency. State Health Complaint Agency.
SHC Law. Laws made by each **SHC Agency** to give effect to the National Code. Each SHC Agency re-wrote the National Code to fit its legal framework. The resulting SHC Laws vary from that set down in the National Code. Some States have added extra obligations.

© O Bruhn 2022

24. Care & Feedback

Elements Of Care

Obtain Prior Informed Consent

Informed Consent at Registration. The client needs to be fully informed about learning Stillness Meditation and be given the opportunity to ask any questions, so they can volunteer consent. Discussions and consent (including for touch) should be expressed in writing and a copy retained. Also refer Ch. 26.

Touch (see Ch. 19). Informed prior consent is provided prior to class attendance in which touch occurs. During Stillness Meditation, the teacher is unable to ask for verbal consent as this would take the client (and others) away from mental Stillness. It would reduce the standard of care. Unlike the black and white use of words, touch involves preverbal communication of feelings (ie. trust and calm). If touch is too soon or too close, it may alert the client. The teacher fine tunes by increasing "the space between" so touch reassures and calms. This process permits, or after adjustment, restores preverbal consent.

Unrelated purposes. Separate consent needs to be obtained for unrelated purposes eg. before recording (eg. photo, audio, video), permitting a third party to observe Stillness Meditation sessions and for mailing lists (it is also necessary to provide a way of opting out). If some other matter comes up, it is best to seek consent from the client (and, if necessary, check with the relevant Agency).

Work Within Your Professional Limits

Provide Stillness Meditation services within experience, training and qualifications. Maintain competencies. Seek guidance from experienced colleagues, if needed. Recognise limitations and refer clients to others, if required.

Minimise Risk of Harm & Provide Timely Help

The teaching of Stillness Meditation and teacher-client relationship has been discussed. Safe daily practice of Stillness Meditation is encouraged. Empathy, reassurance, support, and debriefing are provided. **C F A R** (below) is also appropriate.

Crisis supports. Provide crisis support contacts at registration, so they are accessible to the client (including to help someone else!).

www.lifeline.org.au 131114
www.suicidecallbackservice.org.au 1300659467
www.kidshelp.com.au 1800551800
www.mensline.org.au 1300789978

Reassurance, feedback and support are provided before, during and after Stillness Meditation. Client statements and or behaviour may lead flag concerns. Some instances, may require referral of the client to crisis &/or friendly supports suited to their situation/needs. Check the client has crisis support contacts on their phone. Consider offering or making a crisis report on their behalf, if this seems warranted.

Friendly Supports. These include next-of-kin, carer, relatives and GP. They should be kept informed, so they can provide support.

Assistance. Sometimes, obvious suggestions can be made for obvious problems eg. training; community care; financial, vocational or rehabilitation guidance and so on.

Referral. For example, medical clearance might be needed before teaching unusual clients (see later). Client permission is needed for the teacher to contact another health provider AND for the other provider (ie. AHPRA or not) to discuss the client's health.

Respectful Culturally Sensitive Service

Meditation teachers must respect the values, beliefs, and aspirations of clients together with the trust placed in them by the client. Inclusiveness requires equal treatment that includes diversity within culture. Some specific issues are discussed below.

Non English speaking background. If the client requires a translator then this may also indicate that they might not be able to be taught due to lack of language comprehension. Referral may be needed. Judgement is required.

Severe health disorders. Registration forms should request health history. Those who disclose relevant serious issues such as psychosis, neurological disorders, ageing or acquired brain injury may need to be cleared in writing for Stillness Meditation by their doctor.

Several of these disorders can damage the mechanism(s) that allows Stillness to occur and may also remove capacity for consent. Client (and kin or legally appointed carer, if needed) are informed a trial will reveal if it can be learnt. There might be success or a decision not to pursue that which lies beyond reach.

Religion. People have the right to freedom of thought, conscience, religion and belief. Meares' method is non-religious. It can also be practised alongside a formal religion. Thus, churches may permit Stillness Meditation to be taught on their premises as there is no doctrinal conflict. Atheists and agnostics can also learn Stillness Meditation as it does not contradict their belief system.

Pets in the meditation room would be disruptive and would alarm clients with cynophobia (10%)[169] or allergic to dogs (10%).[170] Assistance dogs help people with disabilities. Seek advice (eg. Human Rights Agency) when balancing the rights of both groups.

Table 1. Working With Children Checks[171]

State	Law	Description	Valid
ACT	Working with vulnerable people Act 2011	Individuals in regulated child related activities must be registered ie. general (transferable), role-based or conditional.	5 yrs
NSW	Child protection (working with children) amendment Act 2018	Individuals apply for certification. Employers verify with NSW Office of Child Guardian that individuals have or have applied for work with children check (WWCC).	5 yrs
NT	Care & protection of children Act 2007	Individuals apply for WWCC 'Ochre Card' aka Clearance Notice.	2 yrs
QLD	Working with children (risk management & screening) Act 2000	Individuals apply for WWCC aka 'Blue Card'. Child-related services must have policies & procedures that minimise risk of harm to children.	3 yrs
SA	Child safety act 2016 Childrens protection Act & Regulations	Employers & responsible authorities must obtain National Police Checks and conduct child-related employment screening for those in child-related occupations/ volunteering.	5 yrs
Tas	Registration to work with vulnerable people Act 2013	Individuals in child-related sectors must apply for Working With Vulnerable People check.	5 yrs
Vic	Worker screening Act 2020	Individuals must apply for WWCC.	5 yrs
WA	Working with children criminal record checking Act 2004	Individuals apply for a WWCC.	3 yrs

Children. Look to the work of Pauline McKinnon and Associates (refer footnote)[172].

Criminal record checks are part of AHPRA and School Teacher registration. Meditation teachers wishing to teach children may need a "Working With Children Check" (see table and its footnote). Even if not required by law, third parties may insist. Kin or carer should

---

169 *10% population approx based on unreferenced data on reputable websites.*
170 https://www.healthdirect.gov.au/cat-and-dog-allergy
171 From: https://aifs.gov.au/cfca/publications/pre-employment-screening-working-children-checks-and-police-checks/part-overview accessed mid 2022.
172 Let's Be Still (Manual: teaching Stillness meditation to children & adolescents)

be present in 1:1 sessions with a minor. If parents are separated or divorced then, all court orders <u>must</u> be sighted and understood before registration can be finalised.

The above subheading list is not comprehensive. If doubt exists, obtain further information and, if needed, medical, legal and or SHC Agency advice.

Clients Encouraged to Inform Doctor

The client is encouraged to inform their doctor about learning Stillness Meditation. The doctor needs to know, so they can factor in changed signs and or symptoms. Medications and dosages may change if the doctor advises this is appropriate (and the patient consents). Meditation Teachers must not advise clients to take (or cease taking) prescribed medications (also see Ch. 25).

Access to Code & Complaint Process

The **National Code**[173] states to the effect that providers must display or make available the <u>Code</u> and information about <u>how clients may complain</u> to the SHC Agency.

On their website, the Vic. SHC Agency states:[174] ***"We are happy to provide the following text you can copy and publish on your health service website should you wish***: *If you are not satisfied with our service, please contact us. We take complaints seriously and aim to resolve them quickly and fairly. If you remain dissatisfied with our response, you may contact the* **SHC AGENCY**. *The* **SHC AGENCY** *responds to complaints about health services and the handling of health information in* **STATE**... *To lodge a complaint with the* **SHC AGENCY** *fill out a complaint form online at* **WEBSITE** *or* **PHONE** *between* **TIME, DAYS** ... *If you want more than 20 copies of ... our Making a Complaint brochure* please email us[175] *Otherwise, you can download each brochure or posters* here for your use[176]*."*

---

173 "*17(1) A health care worker must <u>display or make available</u> a copy of...:*
  a. a copy of this <u>Code of Conduct</u> [AND]
  b. a document that gives information about <u>the way in which clients may make a complaint</u> to... [SHC Agency name].
17(2) Copies of these documents must be <u>displayed or made available</u> in a manner that makes them easily <u>visible or accessible</u> to clients. [underlining added]"
"*... a link to the National Code should be made available on the websites of organisations... unable to display the code... There was general support for this proposal.* Final Report. National Code of Conduct for health care workers. COAG Health Council 2015, pg 29
174 https://hcc.vic.gov.au/providers/general-health-service-providers-code-conduct Accessed 2023-03. *Edited to prompt user to provide needed information.*
175 hcc@hcc.vic.gov.au
176 https://hcc.vic.gov.au/resources/publications

© O Bruhn 2022

Outside of Victoria, use your local SHC Agency format. If it has none, then you might use the above format but do change the Agency name, contact details, web links etc.

Remember, that you also need to make available access to your SHC Agency Code as required by SHC law in your local jurisdiction. The Vict. SHC Agency advised that the Vict Code could be reproduced in this book but should not as it might become out of date and a link to their website would not.

Compliments, Concerns & Complaints

Feedback consists of compliments, concerns, and complaints. The majority of feedback is positive or relates to misunderstandings. These can be remedied once identified.

SHC Agencies have mandatory complaint handling standards[177]. These must be reflected in your policy and approach. In principle, complaint handling includes:
- Informing clients how to raise a concern and how these are handled. That way you will hear about problems before the client gets frustrated or an ongoing problem worsens.
- Concerns may be raised about registration, services, referral, behaviour, communication, privacy/ health information, combinations or other clients (refer Ch 23).
- Prompt acknowledgement and appropriate resolution.
- Keep complainant informed of progress and outcomes.
- Keep complaint information confidential.
- Remedial actions depend on the concerns raised eg. apology, explanation, access or amend health record, refund and so on. An opportunity for improvement may also be identified.
- Record complaint and actions taken. If the client requests a response in writing then this must be provided. A response in writing, even if not required by client, can be produced to the SHC Agency, if needed later on. A carefully written reply removes doubt as to what was said or discussed. SHC Law[178] also requires that your response explains that the client may lodge a complaint with the SHC Agency. You can draw on the general text that you have already used to explain clients may complain to SHC Agency (see previous page).

Some further tips on handling complaints include:
- Obtain advice from professional associations, insurers, SHC

---
[177] Vict:*https://hcc.vic.gov.au/providers/complaint-handling-standards* accessed end 2022

[178] *Vict. Complaint Handling Standard 7: A response to the complainant includes information about how to make a complaint to the HCC. See footnote 168.*

and\or Privacy Agency regarding any unclear or undefined matters. Their advice may help decide the best course of action although it may be "all care and no responsibility".
- Make notes of all discussions with witnesses, client who raised concerns, professional associations, Agencies etc. Without notes, it may be difficult to demonstrate what actually happened or was said.
- Witnesses who can corroborate matters are helpful.
- A person who complains to provider or SHC Agency is protected from victimisation or detriment. Make sure your actions don't resemble these things in hindsight. Or, if that can't be avoided (eg. to comply with SHC Law) you might seek advice (eg. SHC Agency) regarding your proposed action and any necessary supporting actions and or documentation.
- After the Agency has made its own enquiries the Agency may refuse, or cease to deal with complaints that are:
    - Reported without attempt to seek provider resolution.
    - Resolved (due to accepting provider actions).
    - Withdrawn.
    - Misconceived, vexatious, frivolous, false or lacking in substance.
    - Not made in good faith.
    - Made for an improper purpose.

Explaining to each client how to raise a concern or complaint means that you should hear promptly about any concerns (which is helpful). Once the concern is reported it is often a matter of taking simple steps leading to remedial actions eg. apology, explanation, access or amend health record, refund or other remedy. A summary of concern, simple steps and outcome should be recorded. Complexity of case will be reflected in process. Rigorous application will be needed to handle outliers.

It may all sound a bit glum. This is partly due to the fact that most people are unaware of these protocols. Of course, the SHC Agency view is that ignorance is no excuse. So, a little glum now might save much glum later.

25. "Do Nots" & Reporting

Meditation Teacher "Do Nots"

Knowledge of "must nots" helps one to keep distant from situations that might resemble a "must not" in hindsight. Applying what you learn in this chapter helps to add a safety margin.

Ill, Infected or Substance Affected Teacher

Check with your health practitioner that:
- Any conditions you have won't *impair* your ability to teach,
- Any *medications prescribed* won't affect your ability to teach,
- Any transmissible *conditions* can't be passed onto clients,

And if teaching needs to be modified (or stopped) until it is safe to resume. The advice of the correct category of health practitioner is needed, as follows:[179]
- Impairment - "*suitably qualified health practitioner*".
- Prescribed medication - "*prescribing health practitioner or dispensing pharmacist*".
- Transmissable condition - "*qualified registered health practitioner*".

Get the relevant practitioner's advice in writing and keep a copy for your records. Obviously, one must not teach under the influence of unlawful substances or alcohol.

Client Treatment by Other Providers

- Clients should be encouraged to seek medical or other healthcare etc, if needed.
- Don't refuse reasonable cooperation with other providers (see later re: mandatory reporting).
- Don't attempt to dissuade a client from seeking or continuing medical treatment. [NB treatment includes prescribed drugs or substances, therapies etc).
- *DO advise the client of any possible adverse interactions between... [meditation] and any other:*
  - *therapies, treatments, prescribed drugs or substances that the client is taking or receiving.*

---

[179] *Italicised professions as defined in the National Code.*

Some adverse interactions that might come up:
- Ch. 5. see "Non-Stillness – A Cautionary Note"
- Ch. 6. see "Combining Treatments"

The client is informed that:
- You can only summarise possible adverse interactions as you must not dissuade them from medical treatment.
- A further medical opinion can be sought, at their discretion.

Some sensation seeking types take various substances, mostly illegal. Clearly, Stillness Meditation teachers don't suggest taking illegal substances. Dr Meares repeatedly mentions a link between taking illegal substances and severe mental illness.

The client learning Stillness Meditation keeps up medical treatments like taking prescribed drugs. After patient <u>and</u> treating doctor agree the time is right the patient might transition to a reduced dose. Drug dose is a medical matter to which the patient consents and the Stillness Meditation teacher is not directly involved. At the client's request (and consent) the meditation teacher might provide feedback to the doctor about client progress.

Avoid Misleading Clients

Don't mislead clients about products, services, qualifications, training or professional affiliation. False claims must not be made. The SHC Agencies are very concerned about false claims about treating or curing cancer and terminal illnesses. Also, refer Ch.6.

Avoid Inappropriate Relationships

Don't engage in sexual misconduct. A provider must not engage in behaviour of a sexual OR close personal nature with a client. Nor must a provider engage in a sexual OR other inappropriate close personal, physical or emotional relationship with a client.[180] A reasonable duration[181] must elapse after conclusion of the provider client relationship before engaging in a sexual relationship with a former client.

Avoid Financial Exploitation

Only provide services to clients designed to maintain or improve their health or wellbeing. Don't financially exploit them. This includes not offering or accepting financial inducements (or gifts) for referrals. Also, not asking clients to give, lend or bequeath money (or gifts) to you, your family, friends or any entity in which you have an interest.

In the case of trivial gifts, factors like courtesy, cultural

---

180 "other inappropriate... relationship" *is undefined as at end 2022.*
181 *undefined as at end 2022. No explanatory guidance existed in Victoria.*

sensitivity and context means there may be no easy answer.

Mandatory Referral of Another Provider

Meditation teachers speak of, and treat, other providers with respect. Yet, a reasonable belief formed in the course of providing treatment or care that *another provider* has or is placing clients at *serious risk of harm* <u>must</u> be referred to the SHC Agency.

Other Provider Falls Within Definition

Categories of providers are defined by each SHC Agency. There is no list. An indicative list is provided below:
- Providers of :
  - disability, aged care and palliative care services
  - health education services,
  - therapeutic counselling and psychotherapeutic services,
  - "anyone providing a service intended or claimed... to assess, predict, maintain or improve the person's physical, mental or psychological health[182]..."
- Ancillary and support services related to the above.

Other examples include: physical trainers, life coaches, yoga teachers, ski instructors, provider receptionists & admin staff, laundries, disposal services, specimen collection and so on.

Information concerning client work role should be requested at registration. A subsequent change to a client's role may not be known to you, if not mentioned by the client. It is important to update client information, as needed.

If you heard about the other (alleged) harm causing provider from someone who is <u>not</u> a current client then a complaint to the SHC Agency might be considered.

Serious Risk Of Harm

Risk is often defined as probability, possibility or likelihood. Harm is defined as things like: physical and mental damage, injury, reduced value or loss. If unsure, seek advice from SHC Agency.

Elements of a Mandatory Referral

Avoid a knee-jerk response. Work out:
- Is it referable?
  - "*Provider*" falls within definition.
  - Heard about during your own "*providing*".
  - "*Serious risk of harm*" is present.

"Vexatious referrals" are ones with no substance, intended to

---

182 *As at end 2022, Some States had modified these criteria.*

distress or disadvantage the named provider. AHPRA[183] views them as misconduct. An accurate mandatory referral is needed to avoid any potential for the SHC Agency drawing a similar conclusion.

Turning a Blind Eye...

SHC Agency staff investigate complaints and will interview at risk or harmed people. The names of any other providers will be sought. These may be followed up to get evidence they require. Turning a blind eye to another providers harmful actions may create a risk that the SHC Agency turning its gaze in your direction.

Conflicts of Interest

The National Code doesn't mention conflicts of interest. AHPRA and professional association codes invariably mention them. The Meditation Australia Code mentions them.

Avoid any conflict of interest, by declaring and, so far as is workable, take appropriate steps to address them. Solo teachers will be unable to completely avoid all conflicts and this reiterates the importance of declaring them when they arise.

Dual relationships where the teacher interacts with a client separate from teaching can lead to a conflict. This includes slipping between the provider role and: -
- Bartering services with clients.
- Offering payment breaks (ie, becoming a creditor).
- Engaging in a social (platonic) relationship with a client.
- Accepting gifts from clients.
- Going into business with a client.
- Use of social media.

Inappropriate Client Behaviour

Failing to deal with inappropriate client behaviour can lead to a conflict of interest. A first step is to specify behaviours expected of clients that draws a line (see over page). This is provided at registration. The line helps those who need to be reminded and helps identify any crossing into inappropriate behaviour later.

Later on, if concerns were raised, enquiries and checks are needed to ensure you have an accurate understanding, prior to taking action. Review Ch. 24 (complaints). Speak with any witnesses. Review all further sources of information. When you have all the facts, then meet with the acused client and inform them about the concerns. Ensure they are given an oppurtunity to explain. If necessary, seek further new information. The outcomes may include:

---

[183] AHPRA. Code of Conduct for national boards. Jun 2022. pages 21 & 30.

no action (if concerns untrue or trivial), comment, warning, reprimand etc. Suspension or expulsion maybe warranted for serious acts. If a criminal act is likely to have been committed then reporting may be considered (or required). A written summary of your enquiries, findings and action outcomes should be provided to the acused client. It must mention that they can complain to the SHC Agency. The SHC Agency will request it from a complainant as evidence the complaint has been raised with the provider. It might sound gloomy but, careful actions will help to minimise any gloom and let the light in so it shines on whom it should.

Guiding Appropriate Behaviour

Appropriate human behaviour can be facilitated by information, instruction, training and supervision. One aspect of this is providing a set of points or "rules". Contractual agreements and complete specification are beyond the scope of this book as they require consideration of niche audience, setting, provider entity, existance or absence of third parties like venue providers and so on. Legal (not limitd to SHC Agency law) and other elements need to be included.

It is only possible to offer a starting point. The list below is not exhaustive and it will need to be modified to fit your circumstances. Further items may be needed for special applications or to interface with venue provider requirements (eg.evacuation, security cameras, other?).

Always, remember that aids (eg. lists) can have an unintended side effect of acting like a set of blinkers. Think outside the square. The list is just a starting point and is outlined below:

Clients have a right to:
- Respect, courtesy and consideration.
- A supportive environment, free of discrimination and harassment.
- Privacy of personal information held. Confidentiality is to be observed in regard to personal or professional disclosures made by other clients or staff.
- A safe and healthy environment as far as is reasonably practicable.
- Lodge a concern ("complaint") without fear of victimisation.
- Other?

Clients are expected to:
- Arrive a few minutes before the starting time. Each session starts on time. After clients have arrived the teacher closes

- the door(s) and the session commences, late comers cannot join the class.
- Enter and leave class\venue when requested by teaching staff. For OHS, venues have emergency evacuation routes marked on a map displayed by venue.
- Turn off mobile phones\ electronic devices.
- Not move chairs nor use a chair signposted ("reserved") unless advised by teaching staff.
- Stow personal items under seats to avoid creating trip hazards.
- Remove spectacles, hats & heavy jewellery and stow them safely.
- Noise and movement outside the room may occur and are monitored by the teacher. All you need do is to allow the experience of Stillness to unfold.
- Please remain seated at the finish until called by name. When called a private discussion will occur outside the room. You will be invited to discuss any concerns.
- If drowsy after meditation then rest until wide awake. Don't walk in traffic or drive till wide awake!
- Others?

<u>Clients are also expected to</u>:
- Not bring children (or pets) to class (separate childcare is needed).
- Not consume food in class.
- Not smoke tobacco or vape inside or around venue.
- Not be under the influence of alcohol, drugs or unlawful substances.
- Not take photographs, videos or recordings without all parties' consent.
- Not make public statements purporting to be on behalf of the Service.
- After ceasing relationship and or attendance, all trust and confidentiality previously made shall remain binding.
- Others?

26. OHS, Insurance & Records

Occupational Health & Safety (OHS) Law

Providers may be employers, sole traders or contractors. OHS legislation obliges such persons to "as far as reasonably practicable" protect the OHS of employees and people who are not employees (ie. clients and visitors). This may, at times, overlap with duties required by other regulators and associations (see earlier). The focus of OHS relates to the risks and related harm that might occur at workplaces. The scope of OHS is wider than Stillness Meditation teaching as such. The arrangements for one person renting a room on a sessional basis will differ from an entity that employees many people. If you need to further clarify OHS requirements, refer to the website and services of your State OHS Authority:-

ACT www.worksafe.act.gov.au
NSW www.safework.nsw.gov.au
NT www.worksafe.nt.gov.au
Qld www.worksafe.qld.gov.au
SA www.safework.sa.gov.au
Tas www.worksafe.tas.gov.au/
Vic www.worksafe.vic.gov.au
WA www.commerce.wa.gov.au/worksafe
Comcare www.comcare.gov.au

Workplace First Aid

SHC and OHS laws both require first aid, emergency assistance ("000") and later remedial action to prevent recurrence. See Ch. 24 re: crisis support. SHC Law also requires disclosure to the client of an "adverse" event arising during treatment or care.

The Victorian Workplace Compliance Code for First Aid 2021. pg8 requires that a low risk micro-business (eg. office, library and most shops) must have an accessible first aid kit. Such and entity:
- employs less than 10 people,
- not exposed to hazards that may result in serious injury or illness requiring immediate treatment,
- medical or ambulance services are readily available.

If you teach meditation at different locations consider keeping a first aid kit, in your car parked at the venue so it is readily accessible. Out of sight, so not stolen. The kit needs to be kept restocked (see table).

First Aid training is required by some associations. The SHC requires that emergency and first aid is provided rather than specifying training as such (in Victoria, anyway).

Also, be aware that an injury requiring first aid, or emergency assistance, needs to be recorded. It may also need to be reported to either State OHS Agency (ie. if a specified notifiable incident) &/or the SHC Agency *("relevant authority"[184])*.

First Aid Kit Contents
Basic first aid notes
Disposable gloves
Resuscitation mask
Individually wrapped sterile adhesive dressings
Sterile eye pads (packet)
Sterile coverings for serious wounds
Triangular bandages
Safety pins
Small, medium and large sterile unmedicated wound dressings
Non-allergenic tape
Rubber thread or crêpe bandage
Scissors
Tweezers
Book for recording details of first aid provided
Sterile saline solution
Plastic bags for used item storage and safe disposal
Contact details of medical & emergency services in/on first aid kit.
No pain killers (eg. paracetamol) as diagnosis must precede treatment.

Generic Medical Emergency tips
1. Check for threatening situation & control it, if safe to do so
2. Stay with casualty (unless there is no other way to summon aid*)
3. Do not move casualty unless in a life threatening situation
5. Phone 000 for ambulance & designate someone to meet them
6. Provide support to any first aider\ ambulance as required
*Remember: Danger Response Airway Breathing Circulation
*Notify person in charge.

Inspect, Assess Risk, Control & Maintain

Risks can be reduced by risk assessment, regular inspection and maintenance of building, floor surfaces, chairs, electrical equipment etc. to reduce trips, slips or falls etc. Cleaning, personal and workplace hygiene standards need to be maintained.

---

[184] *National Code 5(2)(d) states: "a health care worker must report the <u>adverse event</u> to the <u>relevant authority</u>, where appropriate". Undefined terms underlined.*

Fire

Evacuation may be safer than attempting to put a fire out. It requires notifying emergency services (000), an evacuation signal, a lit safe route out, through doors that can be easily opened (ie. via a single action). The route leads to a prearranged safe assembly point where a head count establishes everyone has got out (records of those attending class are needed and are taken with you to the assembly area). Check doors, lighting and route. Check the route avoids taking people close to other hazards. Avoid crossing roads to get to the assembly point, if possible. Large workplaces and bushfire prone areas will need more complicated arrangements. Your local OHS Authority, fire brigade or council will be able to provide details, including regarding fire extinguishers etc. and additional requirements. In a one person organisation, the meditation teacher is responsible for the design and triggering of the emergency procedure. If you are contracting to another organisation or renting a venue then your procedure may be part of someone elses and may include things like emergency wardens and so on.

Generic evacuation tips
1. Raise Alarm by alerting persons nearby, phoning 000 or by *(insert other pre-arranged actions)*
2. Rescue anyone in danger if safe to do so.
3. Restrict danger area if safe eg. fire - close doors, use extinguisher.
4. Move to assembly point when unsafe to remain in area. (Or, on signal from warden, if they exist and are present).
5. Assist visitors & disabled persons to evacuate.
6. Remain at final assembly point (aka evacuation area) until instructed by warden or emergency personnel.

Building Damage

Major. If major building damage occurs then evacuate and prevent re-entry by locking doors and signage.

Minor. If damage is minor it may be able to be safely isolated by use of barriers and signs etc. Turn off services (eg. gas, water, power), if safe to do so, as needed to achieve further safety.

Other Emergencies

Security concerns may arise during access and egress involving isolated areas, especially after dark. Good lighting, leaving and arriving in groups are examples of common measures. Risk assessment will identify any other risks eg. the risk of unwanted persons accessing the premises during class could be dealt with by "lock-down" (lock doors & windows etc) with emergency services contacts (eg. 000) readily accessible.

Insurance

Public liability and professional indemnity insurance are required by prudence, SHC Law and some professional associations. Compliance with SHC Agency, OHS, Building and Local Council requirements are amongst those conditions that insurers mention.

In 2022, some Australian Insurers offered professional indemnity cover starting at $1 million AUD and public liability starting at $10 million AUD. In 2022, some take out cover for twice those amounts, or more, due to concerns about all potential costs including legal fees being able to be met. Specialist advice that considers the individual Stillness Meditation teachers circumstances will help identify the right amount of cover. Premiums are typically in the hundreds of dollars range. Dollar amounts depend upon individual circumstances, coverage and will change over time.

Individual policies detail what is covered. It is important they include: all categories of events, legal costs and, both current and retrospective events. In other words, events that happened in the past as well as going forwards to the end of the cover. Finding out cover offered for other professionals in similar circumstances may help you choose appropriate and adequate cover for your own.

Insurance company employees are the insurer's agent, not yours. If you feel unsure about cover get advice rather than finding out that a claim is "out of bounds" as well as "out of pocket".

Records & Privacy

Keep Records, Comply With Privacy Law

Maintain accurate, legible and up-to-date records for each client that are secured to prevent unauthorised access.

Facilitate client access or transfer their record if requested by the client (or legal representative).

Record complaints. Below is a brief outline of the Health Record Privacy Principles:

1. Collect health information (HI), with consent, needed for a specified primary purpose. Ensure client knows why it is collected and how it is handled.
2. Use and disclose HI for a primary or directly related purpose and only for another purpose with consent (unless authorised by law).
3. Take reasonable steps to ensure HI is accurate, complete, up-to-date and relevant to functions performed.
4. Store HI securely, protecting HI from unauthorised access.
5. Retain HI for period authorised by statutes of limitation.
6. Provide the client with access to HI and the right to seek its correction.

© O Bruhn 2022

7. If a provider's practice is being sold, transferred or closed down give notice of transfer or closure to past clients.
8. Make HI available to another provider on client request.
9. Provide the client your documented policy on managing HI on request.

Commonwealth (Cth) and State Privacy Laws are based on these Privacy Principles. The relevant laws are outlined in the table below. If a State has no health record privacy law then the Commonwealth law automatically applies (as set out in the table below).

	Public Sector	Private Sector
Cth*	Privacy Act 1988 (Cth) Freedom of Information Act 1982 (Cth)	Privacy Act 1988 (Cth)
ACT	Health Records (Privacy & Access) Act 1997	Privacy Act 1988 (Cth)
NSW	Health Records & Information Privacy Act 2002	Health Records & Info Privacy Act 2002
Vic	Freedom of Information Act 1982	Health Records Act 2001
NT	Information Act	Privacy Act 1988 (Cth)
Qld	Information Privacy Act 2009 Right to Information Act 2009	Privacy Act 1988 (Cth)
Tas	Right to Information Act 2009 Personal Information & Protection Act 2004	Privacy Act 1988 (Cth)
SA	Freedom of Information Act 1991	Privacy Act 1988 (Cth)
WA	Freedom of Information Act 1992	Privacy Act 1988(Cth)

If unsure, or complex privacy concerns are raised, then ask the regulator. The relevant websites are listed below:

Clth www.oaic.gov.au (Commonwealth)   ACT hrc.act.gov.au/health
NSW www.ipc.nsw.gov.au   NT infocomm.nt.gov.au
Qld www.oic.qld.gov.au & www.oho.qld.gov.au
Tas www.ombudsman.tas.gov.au   Vic www.hcc.vic.gov.au
WA www.oic.wa.gov.au

Generic Protocol Referencing Records

This is list is generic. Additional elements may be needed for special applications.

Prior to registration - information provided by teacher
Biography – story and meditation experience (Ch. 18).
Qualifications & professional memberships (Ch. 25).
Scope of services.
Prior to (or at) registration - request
Referral letters (usually "clearance" letters), if required. (Ch. 24)
At registration
  Provide:
Scope of services & disclaimers.

Crisis support contacts (Ch. 24)
Privacy Policy (Ch. 26)
Feedback & Complaint protocol incl SHC Law standards (Ch. 24).
Access to SHC Agency version of National Code (see Ch. 24).
Refund & cancellation policy eg. teacher ill, alternative classes etc.
Inappropriate client behaviour policy (Ch. 25).
Mandatory referral policy (Ch. 25).
Payment ie. pay/session or pay for bundled sessions.

Obtain:

Birth date, address, emergency contacts, GP, occupation (Ch. 24).
Any critical health advice for paramedics.
Reason(s) for learning Stillness Meditation.
Health History volunteered by client.
Consent for treatment & touch (Ch. 24).
If needed, signed consent to communicate with other health providers about client's health information. Release signed by client, so the other provider is able to reply. (Sign off is needed for all "**provide**" and "**obtain**" matters).

Ongoing records:

Plan and response to Stillness Meditation.
Dates and times of classes\appointments.
Notes taken after each class (often may say "OK" or similar etc).
Notes taken in the event of any incident (eg. crisis support, complaints, inappropriate treatment by other provider etc).
Any letters/reports to and from other professionals.
Fees paid and outstanding.

Destruction of records

Generally, the records of 18+ yo clients need to be kept for 7 years from time of last contact. For a minor (last contact <18 yrs), records must be kept until after 25yo. These times override any requests by client to dispose of records. Do check requirements with your local jurisdiction.

Records disposal must destroy or permanently de-identify personal information. A **register of destroyed records** should be kept that includes client name, periods of time records covered and date(s) of destruction. A file destruction company may be used. It needs to conform with confidential field destruction standards and provide certificates that covers the destroyed documentation. The certificate needs to be retained and contain the same information as the destroyed records register would have done.

© O Bruhn 2022

27. Fees & Sources of Advice

Fees

The setting of fees needs to consider:
- The time involved both inside and outside of class.
- Utilisation rate (eg. paid 30% of week ie. 10 hours).
- How much income you earn per hour (ie. plus all costs).
- Whether the teaching is consultation or charity.

In the world of "general" consultants, work is viewed as billable hours (or utilisation rate) plus the rest. They say they work full time from which you infer they are paid 40+ hrs/week. Privately, they hope that billable hours are 50% of work hours. 50% doubles the hourly rate sought. 33% utilisation triples it.

Some thought about fees is necessary as no one can operate for long at a loss. Knowing class size, costs (administration, venue, utility, professional costs [memberships, insurance, professional development etc] and utilisation rate helps to calculate the break even point - no loss but no profit either. This will help set viable fees.

Competitors rates (eg. yoga & other health modalities), per head in class and solo, are a consideration in fee setting. Fees should also reflect the value perceived by clients. Comparisons might include the cost of going to movies, eating out, spectator sports, a haircut, trades person attendance etc. Offering overly low cost services may send the wrong signal. Stillness Meditation offers a very high level of service via a qualified teacher, touch and small class size. In general, Meditation Australia suggests:[185]

$100-150/hr	1 to 1
$240-500/hr	Community Group\ School
$600—1000+/hr	Corporate

The rates finally agreed are those that clients are willing to pay and that the teacher is comfortable charging.

Teaching may be full time, part time or a side line. Consider transitioning in stages eg. a part-time teaching startup that expands in stages at the same as other work is reduced. This helps provide income stability and allows some slack for learning.

There may be strengths in spreading your eggs in more than one basket eg. teaching at 2-3 venues, in case a spot is lost. Alternatively,

---

185 https://meditationaustralia.org.au/membership/suggested-pricing/ accessed end 2022.

a long term arrangement secures a venue for a longer time. Best to make sure the venue, neighbours, other tenants and so on are suitable, if you decide to go down that track. Some rental /lease agreements have termination (and other) penalties. Advisers may be able to identify further advantages and pitfalls (see below).

Sources of Further Advice

These include:
- Pay and conditions www.fairwork.gov.au
- Income tax and GST www.ato.gov.au
- Copyright www.copyright.org.au
- Environment www.epa.vic.gov.au (Vic)

States governments and some local councils also have resources:
ACT www.act.gov.au/economic-support
NSW www.nsw.gov.au/working-and-business
NT nt.gov.au/industry/start-run-and-grow-a-business
Qld www.business.qld.gov.au   Tas www.business.tas.gov.au
SA business.sa.gov.au   Vic www.business.vic.gov.au
WA www.wa.gov.au/service/business-support

A final option is to access the services of business advisers like an accountant or lawyer. Fee-for-service advice from specialists is an option to consider particularly for difficult problems or where your own resources are to be limited to Stillness Meditation teaching. Some people get help to set up systems themselves, run them and then get input later to identify any improvements. These choices are available but further discussion is beyond the scope of this book.

Accountants

Chartered Accountants ANZ (CA) www.charteredaccountantsanz.com
Institute of Public Accountants (IPA)   www.publicaccountants.org.au
Cert. Practising Accountants Aust (CPA) www.cpaaustralia.com.au

There is nothing to stop anyone from calling themselves an accountant. Use the links to check your choice is a member of one or more of the organisations above and is a CA, IPA or CPA.

Lawyers

ACT www.actlawsociety.asn.au   NSW www.lawsociety.com.au
NT lawsocietynt.asn.au   Qld www.qls.com.au
SA www.lawsocietysa.asn.au   Tas members.lst.org.au

Vic www.liv.asn.au   WA www.lpbwa.org.au
State legal societies have find-a-lawyer searches to identify those currently entitled to practice by postcode and topic expertise.

https://www.nationallegalaid.org/contact/ lists State Legal Aid contacts who <u>may</u> provide limited free legal advice. Their services are triaged towards the socially and economically disadvantaged.

S6. Afterwards

28. Meares' Article Bibliography

Some points to help use the bibliography:
- Meares' books are listed and contents of each summarised in <u>A Key to the Books of Ainslie Meares</u>.
- Journal articles are in plain text.
- Footnotes explain:
  - If an article was written much earlier than the publication date.
  - Some citation errors seen in other sources.
- Symbols flag articles in the following categories:
  - \# Teaching
  - * Cancer
  - ^ Pain management

1954

Defences against hypnosis. Brit J Med Hyp (Spring 1954) pp. 1–6.
Hypnography—a technique in hypnoanalysis. J Mental Sci. 100(421): 965-974. (*An abridged version was published in the Digest of Neurol & Psychiatry, Feb 1955*).
History-taking and physical examination in relation to subsequent hypnosis. Int J Clin Exp Hyp 2(4): 291-5.
Rapport with the patient. Lancet 264(6838):592-4.
Rapport with the patient. Lancet, 264(6844):921 (*reply to letter*).
The clinical estimation of suggestibility. Int J Clin Exp Hyp 2(2): 106-8.
Non-verbal suggestion in the induction of hypnosis. Br J Med Hyp (Summer) pp. 1–4.
Extra-verbal suggestion in the induction of hypnosis. Brit J Med Hyp (Autumn) pp.1–4.

1955

Anxiety reactions in hypnosis. Brit Med J 1(4928): 1454-8.
A note on the motivation for hypnosis. Int J Clin Exp Hypnosis. 3(4): 222-8.
A dynamic technique for the induction of hypnosis. Med J Aust 1(18): 644-6.

1956
A note on hypnosis and the mono-symptomatic psychoneurotic. Brit J Med Hyp V8(2):2–4.
The hysteroid aspects of hypnosis. Am J Psychiatry 112(11): 916-918. (*An abridged version was published in* Digest of Neurol & Psychiatry, *Jun 1956*).
Non-specific suggestion. Brit J Med Hyp 7(2):16-9.
On the nature of suggestibility. Brit J Med Hyp (Sum 1956) 7: 3–8.
Recent work in hypnosis and its relation to general psychiatry. Pt 1 & Pt 2. Med J Aust 1(1):1-5 & 1(2):37–40.
Truth drugs. Proc Medico-Legal Society Victoria vii pp. 137-151.

1957
A working hypothesis as to the nature of hypnosis. AMA Archiv Neurol & Psychiatry, 77(5): 549-55.
A contribution to medical hypnosis (<u>Doctoral Dissertation</u>, University of Melbourne). *Meares' thesis consists of the journal articles 1954-1957 (excluding the "monosymptomatic psychoneurotic" and "truth drug" articles).*

1958
Hypnosis: an evaluation of its place in medicine. Med J Aust. 45(26): 857-858. [*Paper read at 10th Aust Medical Congress*].

1959
Pills, pain and personality[186]. J World Fed Mental Health. 4: 158-9.
The diagnosis of prepsychotic schizophrenia. Lancet 273(7063):55-8.

1960
Communication with the patient. Lancet. 275(7126): 663-667. [*A summary of this article was in Med Journal Aust 1960 Pt1&2. 1(20):777-778 1(22): 855-856. The Lancet article is referenced.*]
The y-state-an hypnotic variant. Int J Clin Exp Hyp. 8(4): 237-41.

1961
Recognising the schizophrenic before he is psychotic. Consultant. August 1961. pp4-8.
Chhina GS, **Meares A**[187] & Anand BK & Singh B (1961). EEG activity under hypnotism. Ind J Physiol Pharmacol. 5(1):43-8.
An evaluation of the dangers of medical hypnosis. Am J Clin Hyp. 4(2): 90-7.
The atavistic theory of hypnosis in relation to yoga and the pseudo-

---

[186] *Published under the name* Ainslie Mears.
[187] *The work reported was undertaken when Meares was in India in 1960.*

trance states. Pp 712-4. In Proc 3rd World Congress of Psychiatry. Montreal. 1961.
Phychiatric"[188] art and the occupational therapist. Aust Occup Therapy J 13(1): 2-6.
What makes the patient better? Lancet. 1961 Jun 10; 1(7189):1280-1

1962

An atavistic theory of hypnosis, pp73–103 in Kline, MV (Ed). The Nature of Hypnosis: Contemporary Theoretical Approaches, Trans 1961 Int Congress Hypnosis.
Theories of hypnosis in pp390–405 in Schneck, JM (Ed) Hypnosis in Modern Medicine. 1962.[189]
What makes the patient better? Atavistic regression as a basic factor. Lancet. 1962 Jan 20;1(7221):151-3.
What makes the patient better? Can Med Assoc J. 86(14): 665.
The atavistic theory of hypnosis. Med J Aust. 1(19): 711-714. *Paper also delivered at Int Soc Clin Exp Hypnosis Conf. Rio De Janiero 1961. Also, Int Congress on Hypnosis NY 1961.*

1963

What makes the patient better? Lancet 281(7295): 1380-81.

1966

Supraconscious experience. Am J Psychiatry 122(8): 953-4.
#Anxiety and hypnosis. Med J Aust 1(10): 395-7. *Also, read at Int Congress Hyp & Psychosomatic Med. Paris. 1965.*

1967

Consciousness and the atavistic theory of hypnosis. pp32-41 in Kline, MV (Ed). Psychodynamics and hypnosis.[190]
Anxiety and Hypnosis pp217-224 in Lasner J (ed) Hypnosis and psychomatic medicine. Proc Int Congress Hypnosis and Psychosomatic Medicine. France. 1965.[191]
^Psychological control of organically determined pain. Annals Aust College Dent Surg 1:42-6.
Suggestion, hypnosis and intuition. Proc Medico-Legal Society Vict V11: 73-84.
^Pain and the psychiatrist. ANZ J Psychiatry 1(3): 116-7.

---

188 *Spelling was "phychiatric". Librarians deserve more recognition than they get. They worked hard to help me find this article. Sources reference it to 1966 but it is 1961. Printers or proofers misspelled psychiatric as phychiatric.*
189 *This article is in the 3rd Ed Schneck as the article references* Medical System of Hypnosis *and other material that dates to 1961-1962.*
190 *Written in 1964. Meares writes "3 years ago I spent time in India, Burma…."*
191 *Written 2 years earlier in 1965 prior to attending conference.*

^Teaching the patient control of organically determined pain. Med J Aust. 1(1): 11-2.
#The space between. Int J Clin Exp Hyp 15(4):156-9. D*elivered Int Congress Psychosomatic Med & Hypnosis, Japan, July 1967.*

1968
^Psychological Mechanisms in the Relief of Pain by Hypnosis. Am J Clin Hyp 11(1):55-57. D*elivered Int Congress Psychosomatic Med & Hypnosis, Kyoto, Japan, July 1967.*
#Hypnotherapy without the phenomena of hypnosis. Int J Clin Exp Hyp. 16(4):211-4.
"Umm". Med J Aust 2(15): 638.

1969
Matheson JAL (1969) Student protest. Proc Medico-Legal Soc Vict pp283-295. Meares' comments are on pp293-5.
Hypnosis and transcendental religious experience. Existential Psychiatry[192]. pp119-121.
Thoughts of an idle evening. Med J Aust 1(16): 822-3.

1971
The nature, use and abuse of hypnosis. Aust J Forensic Sci 3(4): 157-161. *Read at 11th Plenary Session Aust Acad Forensic Sci. Sydney. March 1971.*
#Group relaxing hypnosis. Med J Aust. 2(13): 675-6. *Read at Int Meeting of Amer Ontoanalytic Assoc. Nov 1970.*

1972
#Group relaxing hypnosis. J Am Soc Psych Dent Med 19(4):137-41. *Reprinted from 1971 Med J Aust article.*

1973
#A psychiatric experiment in community service. Med J Aust 1(15):733-4.
Nervous tension in professional life. Proc Medico-Legal Soc Vict V12:277-284.

1974
The drop out syndrome. Aust Family Physician 3:164-168.

1975
#The reduction of anxiety by autohypnotic meditative experience in non-medical groups pp110-112 in <u>Unestahl LE (Ed). Hypnosis in the seventies. VIth Int Congress for Hypnosis.</u>

---

192 *Written in 1967. Journal of the American Ontoanalytic Assoc. was Existential Psychiatry at that time.*

Hypnosis in relation to meditation, yoga and prayer. pp159-160 in Unestahl LE (Ed). Hypnosis in the seventies. VIth Int Congress for Hypnosis.

1976
#The relief of anxiety through relaxing meditation. Aust Fam Physician 5(7):906-10.
*Regression of cancer after intensive meditation. Med J Aust 2(5):184.

1977
*Atavistic regression as a factor in the remission of cancer. Med J Aust 2(4):132-3.
*Regression of cancer after intensive meditation followed by death. Med J Aust 2(11):374-5.

1978
*Regression of osteogenic sarcoma metastases associated with intensive meditation. Med J Aust 21(9):433-433.
*#The quality of meditation effective in the regression of cancer. J Am Soc Psych Dent Med 25(4):129-32.
*#Vivid visualisation and dim visual awareness in the regression of cancer in meditation. J Am Soc Psych Dent Med 25(3):85-88.

1979
*Mind and cancer. Lancet. May 5. 1(8123): 978[193]
*Meditation and cancer. Yoga Quarterly 14(4):27-32.
*Regression of cancer of the rectum following intensive meditation. Med J Aust 2(10):539-40.
*Meditation: A psychological approach to cancer treatment. The Practitioner. 222(1327): 119-22.
*The psychological treatment of cancer. Aust Fam Physician 8(7):801-5.
*Atavistic communication by touch in the psychological treatment of cancer by intensive meditation. J Holistic Health 4:120-124.

1980
*Remission of massive metastasis from undifferentiated carcinoma of the lung associated with intensive meditation. J Am Soc Psych Dent Med 27(2):40-1.
*What can the cancer patient expect from intensive meditation? Aust Fam Physician. May 9(5):322-5.
*Our attitude of mind in the psychological treatment of cancer. Aust

---

[193] *Article sometimes incorrectly cited with co-authors (Horrobin, Ghayur & Karmali) who wrote a separate article printed on same page as Meares' article.*

Nurses J. 9(7):29-30.
*Massage as an adjunct to meditation in the psychological treatment of cancer. Aust J Physio 26(1):25-6.
*The on-flow of meditation in the psychological treatment of cancer. J Helen Vale Foundation 2(4):10-14.

1981
*Regression of recurrence of carcinoma of the breast of mastectomy site associated with intensive meditation. Aust Fam Physician. 10(3):218-19.
*Cancer, psychosomatic illness and hysteria. Lancet. Nov 7, 2(8254):1037-8.

1982
*Stress, meditation and the regression of cancer. The Practitioner. 226(1371):1607-8.
*Meditation and the prevention of the recurrence of cancer. J Helen Vale Foundation. 3(2): 13-16.
#*A form of intensive meditation associated with the regression of cancer. Am J Clin Hyp 25(2/3):114-21.

1983
*Psychological mechanisms in the regression of cancer. Med J Aust 1(12):583-584.
*Cancer and stress: is meditation the answer? Winthrop Impulse 22(6) Apr pp1-2.

1985
*Counselling the terminally ill. Cancer Forum G(3):88

30. Ongoing Development Tips

Participation in Professional Associations

Meares was actively involved in professional associations (including office bearing positions). He was also a reviewing editor for decades on at least one international journal.

On the way to or from medical conferences, Meares went on field trips to meet with "experts" (yogis, sufis, mystics, etc). from all the major branches of hypnosis, meditation and mysticism present on planet earth. With care, one can learn and not have one's understanding confused or diluted by professional association related activities.

Continuing Supplementary Education

Meares had 2 degrees and postgraduate training. He wrote 36 books and many articles. Roughly a book and several articles each year for most of his career. Partly, development and partly disseminating his method as wide as possible.

Ongoing modern development might include things like mental health first aid or other "micro credentials". Additional skills in counselling or similar disciplines might be helpful but must be kept separate from Stillness Meditation by appropriate sequence and separation (see Ch. 15, 16 & 22).. These added skills could be via taking individual subjects, micro credentialed courses or formal course work.

Mutual Support & Mentoring

Mentoring involves one seeking advice, learning, and support from a more experienced one. Mentoring is an ongoing social learning relationship that benefits both parties. The idea presupposes differing levels between two participants. In many cases, "mentoring" involves mutual learning and support.

Revisit Being a Client

If there are other Meares' Stillness Meditation teachers' nearby one might be able to arrange to occasionally participate in one of their classes. This enables one to experience, as a client, the process adopted by another teacher at another venue. It will be "same but different". I am lucky to have participated in classes run by quite a few different teachers at different locations. Both myself and this book have benefitted from these experiences.

Supplements

If Stillness Meditation and Onflow are the main dish then the supplements (including meditation support factors), are the side dish or spices. Reading Meares' books published after 1967 will allow you to pick up the framework that way. The main elements are "catalogued" in Still Mind Sound Body.

The Discipline of Ease

"By practicing mental relaxation in circumstances of discomfort we train our mind to be at ease when we are faced with the discomforts of daily life... [Things like] physical discomfort, sudden unexpected and chronic pain as well as mental pain like anguish, sorrow, humiliation, guilt".[194]

This training within Stillness Meditation, retains our sensitivity and does not involve masochism. The effortless relaxation that allows the mind to transcend slight discomfort can be made more general by gradually incrementally adding further stimulus during Stillness Meditation. Meares trained this way and was able to effortlessly relax and transcend the discomfort of having several decayed teeth and a sebaceous cyst on his neck removed without anaesthetic on different occassions .[195]

Someone once said to me that emotional and spiritual discomfort are needed for personal growth. I realised that more should be mentioned about the importance of the effortless transcendence of discomfort to make the Stillness more general in meditation. The postural progression begins this process. Then, later on stimuli can be added to Stillness Meditation practice outside the classroom.[196] We learn effortless transcendence of discomfort, which helps us learn to be at ease in daily living, even in situations we used to find difficult.

---

194 Meares A (1978). The Wealth Within. Ch.6 & 7.
195 McCay AR (1963) Med. J. Aust. pg 820; Meares A (1978). The Wealth Within. Ch.6 & 7. Also refer Ainslie Meares on Meditation.
196 Refer previous footnote.

Long have I known the Stillness
Of meditation
But now there comes
A greater Stillness
That does not seem to be
Of mine own self

Silent
As in the autumn
When a falling leaf
Reverberates
The dry leaves on which it falls[197]

---

197 Meares A. Prayer and Beyond. 1981.pg4.

© O Bruhn 2022

www.ingramcontent.com/pod-product-compliance
Lightning Source LLC
Chambersburg PA
CBHW022016290426
44109CB00015B/1183